How Nine Months' Influence Can Last a Lifetime

OBESITY—too little food early in pregnancy may program the fetus' brain so that it triggers overeating in adulthood.

DIABETES—inadequate nutrition may compel the fetus to save and store glucose rather than burn it for fuel, leading to diabetes.

HEART DISEASE—babies born full term but underweight may have an increased chance of developing cardiovascular disease decades later.

HIGH CHOLESTEROL—poor nourishment may lead to a small liver, which then can't clear cholesterol efficiently.

CANCER—a very high birth weight may prime a female's mammary tissue for breast cancer.

SCHIZOPHRENIA—early gestational malnutrition has been found to double the risk of schizophrenia in adulthood.

ASTHMA—low birth weight seems to predispose newborns to asthma later in life.

The Gift of Health

The Complete Pregnancy Diet for Your Baby's Wellness–From Birth Through Adulthood

Karin B. Michels, ScD, MSc, MPH
Assistant Professor of Obstetrics, Gynecology
and Reproductive Biology,
Harvard Medical School

and Kristine Napier, MPH, RD, LD
Nutrition and Culinary Consultant,
Cleveland Clinic Preventive Cardiology Program

Produced by The Philip Lief Group, Inc.

POCKET BOOKS
New York London Toronto Sydney Singapore

All recipes except Celery and Apple Salad, Cucumber Salad, Karin's Banana Breakfast Frappe, and Karin's Müsli, Copyright © 2001 by Kristine Napier, MPH, RD, LD.

Recipes for Western Omelet, Apple Oatmeal, Poppyseed Salmon Salad, Cheesy Spinach Pizza, Rotini Chicken Salad with Peanut Sauce, and Mandarin Breakfast Broil, reprinted by permission of Simon & Schuster from THE XENICAL ADVANTAGE by John Foreyt and Kristine Napier. Copyright © 1999 by The Philip Lief Group, Inc. and John Foreyt.

An *Original* Publication of POCKET BOOKS

 POCKET BOOKS, a division of Simon & Schuster, Inc.
1230 Avenue of the Americas, New York, NY 10020

Copyright © 2001 by The Philip Lief Group and Karin B Michels

ISBN: 0-7434-0749-0

First Pocket Books trade paperback printing August 2001

10   9   8   7   6   5   4   3   2   1

POCKET and colophon are registered trademarks of Simon & Schuster, Inc.

Interior design by Stratford Publishing Services, Inc.

Printed in the U.S.A.

Dedication

For my mother, Erika Maria Elisabeth Michels,
who taught me all about nutrition
—Karin B. Michels

Acknowledgments

My interest in the fetal origins of chronic disease was sparked and fostered through the stimulating discussions with many distinguished scientists around the globe who have dedicated much of their research to this area. Knowledge has advanced through the contributions of all of them. I am grateful to my colleagues for pushing the field of early life risk factors for chronic disease forward, and for the opportunity for scientific exchange, in particular with Anders Ekbom, Dimitrios Trichopoulos, Walter Willett, David Barker, Diana Kuh, Yoav Ben-Shlomo, George Davey Smith, David Leon, Bianca DeStavola, Janet Rich-Edwards, Stephen Buka, and Ezra Susser.

My special thanks goes to my coauthor Kristine Napier, culinary wizard and skilled writer, who has taken great care in compiling the most nutritious meals for expectant moms. Her theme has been to combine optimal nutrient content with delicious taste. If you think healthy food may be bland and boring, you are in for a surprise—Kris's recipes are gourmet meals loaded with the best nutrients mother nature's bounty has to offer.

Thanks to Judy Linden and Fiona Hinton at the Philip Lief Group, who never ceased to encourage me and offer advice. I have been impressed with their dedication to this book, with their insight into the research and nutrition, and with their superb editorial talents. They have contributed significantly to the growing of this book and have made its production as efficient as possible.

I am grateful to Pocket Books for agreeing to publish this book. My editor, Emily Bestler, has been instrumental in the process of developing this book from an idea, and her professional experience combined with her understanding of pregnant women's needs have provided invaluable guidance along the way.

My warm gratitude goes to Robert L. Barbieri, MD, chairman of the Department of Obstetrics, Gynecology and Reproductive Biology at Brigham and Women's Hospital in Boston, for writing the excellent foreword to this book. He combines the talents of a dedicated physician and an exemplary scientist with a vision, and I am grateful for his support of my research ideas and goals.

I owe Walter C. Willett, MD, DrPH, chairman of the Department of Nutrition at Harvard School of Public Health, who has been a source of inspiration and a privilege to work with for many years. His enthusiasm for trying to unveil the role of diet in chronic disease has advanced the field of nutritional epidemiology tremendously.

My research would not be possible without the support of all my colleagues at Harvard University; I especially appreciate having had the opportunity to visit and collaborate with some of the brightest minds at several universities around the world.

I am particularly indebted to Drs. Walter Willett, Alexander M. Walker, and Robert Barbieri for encouraging me to write this book.

—Karin B. Michels

Just as a baby grows from a mere thought between two people, nourished by the warmth and security of mom, this book has grown from the thoughts and nourishment of many people. I thank first of all my co-author, Karin Michels, for her thoughts and expertise which have brought this field to the fore. I am extremely indebted to my electronic wizard, Sara Stuhan, without whom this book would never have made it from Cleveland to other parts of the world where it was needed. I also thank my culinary assistants, Nancy Morgan and Lu Collins—who helped convert my culinary thoughts into food on your plate. Last—but not least—to Judy Linden and Fiona Hinton, whose editorial expertise is unprecedented.

—Kris Napier

Contents

TWO

From Heart Disease to Diabetes: The Impact of Diet and Other Factors on Specific Diseases   38

THREE

Goals, Objectives, and Calories . . . Calories . . . Calories: The Optimal Pregnancy Diet   57

FOUR

The Don't-Miss-It Overview: The Optimal Pregnancy Diet   72

FIVE
The Prepregnancy Optimal Diet   103

SIX
The First-Trimester Optimal Diet   128

SEVEN
The Second-Trimester Optimal Diet   158

EIGHT
The Third-Trimester Optimal Diet   183

Foreword

Every expectant mother wants to ensure that she does everything possible to maximize the health of her baby. Medical researchers have known for decades that diet, lifestyle factors (for example, cigarette smoking), and maternal disease can influence the health of a baby at birth. However, it has only recently become clear that conditions in the womb may affect a child's future risk of adult diseases, including breast cancer, diabetes, obesity, asthma, heart disease, high blood pressure, and psychiatric and behavioral disorders. It is a remarkable medical discovery that the environment in the womb might be an important determinant of a child's risk of developing chronic diseases sixty years into his or her life! In this book, Dr. Karin Michels provides a readable and thorough account of the development of these exciting new findings and then explains how women can use these scientific insights to help ensure their baby's health at birth and well into adulthood.

Why did it take so long for medical science to arrive at the fundamental discovery that conditions in the womb affect a child's long-term risk of adult disease? One major barrier to this finding was that the length of time between what scientists call the "initial causal event" (in this case, the environment in the womb) and the "critical outcome variable" (for instance, the development of breast cancer sixty years after birth) is much longer than the career of a single scientist and therefore is very difficult to study. Another key problem was that the technology needed to accurately assess the environment within the womb (high-quality ultrasonography, advanced laboratory measurements) have been developed and refined only within the last fifteen years. Finally, the scientists with the right set of research skills just weren't focused on this particular problem. It is indeed fortunate that scientists of the caliber of Karin Michels have dedicated their research careers to the further exploration of this important issue.

Scientists who focus on discovery research are like ace detectives. These investigators often sense, or reason through, the solution to a complex problem before anyone else. Sometimes their insights are so amazing that they need to spend considerable time collecting additional clues and facts to prove their solution to their skeptical colleagues. One of Sherlock Holmes's most remarkable skills was his ability to solve a mystery well before anyone else. At times, it seemed Holmes required more time to convince his colleagues of the mystery's solution than it took him to arrive at his solution in the first place! A similar phenomenon exists in science, where a truly remarkable discovery often requires considerable time to achieve acceptance within the scientific community.

This book provides a fascinating look at the key scientific findings pertaining to the impact of conditions in the womb on a child's adult health. It then uses these insights to build a sensible, easy-to-implement series of dietary recommendations to maximize the health of the prenatal environment for both mother and child. These recommendations include an examination of an expectant mother's and her baby's unique needs during the beginning, middle and end of pregnancy. The importance of maintaining calorie levels and getting enough nutrients, especially vitamin B_6, protein, calcium, folic acid, zinc, and iron receive special attention. Specific dietary advice and simple-to-follow meal plans are provided throughout the book as practical examples of how these ideas can be translated into everyday practice.

In my over twenty years as an OB/GYN, I've seen hundreds of expectant mothers who eagerly look for advice that can help them promote the well-being of their babies-to-be. If you are pregnant or are planning to become pregnant, I urge you to read this helpful guide. You'll immediately realize that today, more than ever before, you are uniquely positioned to adopt diet and lifestyle behaviors that can influence conditions in the womb and that may, in turn, also promote the health of your newborn, both as a child and as an adult. I wholeheartedly recommend *The Gift of Health*.

Robert Barbieri, MD
Chair, Department of Obstetrics,
Gynecology and Reproductive Biology
Brigham and Women's Hospital

In the Beginning

The Origins of Our Health

Every morning when I wake up I know that my day will be filled with thoughts and concerns about pregnant women and the future health of their babies-to-be. But it wasn't always this way. Rather than looking at the beginning of new life, I started out focusing on a terrible disease that can take life.

As a woman, a daughter, a sister, *and* a researcher of chronic disease, I was frustrated. I had dedicated my life's work to finding the reason why one particularly dreaded disease, breast cancer, strikes so many women for no apparent cause. *After all, my mom, my grandmothers, my aunts, any one of my three sisters, or I could get this devastating disease, even though it doesn't run in our family.* As medical professionals, my colleagues and I know so much about so many diseases, yet we just weren't coming up with any good clues as to why breast cancer occurs. We couldn't predict who it would strike next.

Yes, genetics plays a role in some cases, but not very many. Only about 5% to 10% of the women struck with breast cancer have a family history—a mother, sister, aunt, or grandmother who had the disease. Similarly, genetic mutations in the breast cancer susceptibility gene BRCA1/BRCA2 are found only in about 5% of women with breast cancer. For the remaining women who get breast cancer, the cause is unknown.

SEARCHING FOR CLUES

As with any disease, finding the reason *why* it occurs is the first step in finding out how to prevent it from ever happening—and in determining

1

strategies to treat or cure it once it occurs. This is what my field of epidemiology, my profession, is all about. We are detectives, trying to connect the dots between a disease and its cause. This means following the trails of many leads, hoping that at least one takes us to a solid clue.

But it was just a few years into my chosen life's work that I realized that I (and my colleagues in the field) were pursuing cold trails. Breast cancer research was stagnating. The only factors we had found that seemed consistently related to the incidence of breast cancer were age itself (our risk of most diseases rises with age), the age at which a woman had her first child, how many children she had early in life, and the ages at which her periods started and ended. In short, our research had taught us that women who have a number of children at a young age are less likely to get breast cancer. For example, a woman who has two children by the time she is twenty years of age is less likely to get breast cancer than a woman who waits to have children until a little later in life or one who doesn't have children at all. *But it just isn't practical to encourage women to change their age of childbearing or to have more children than they were planning to have—to prevent disease.* How could we tell a woman to have two, three, or four children by the time she was twenty? This wasn't a solution we, as women, could live with. And the age at which one's menstruation begins and ends is not something that can be easily changed.

So I made myself go back to square one. *I must be overlooking something,* I thought to myself. I sat down with my basic science books to make sure I hadn't forgotten the details about how cancer affects breast cells. I even took myself back to my medical school studies to renew my understanding of breast tissue itself. Maybe this would point me down a new path in my search.

As I dug deep into the literature on breast tissue, the cells that form it, and the substances that can affect those cells, I focused anew on something I had known since my first days of studying breast cancer but had pushed to the side somehow. The well-known facts grabbed my attention with such force that I felt as if I were reading it for the first time.

Here's what caught my attention like the 6 o'clock news: breast tissue is one of the most sensitive tissues in the body. More than any other place in the body, the cells in the breast react very strongly to the body's own naturally produced chemicals. Hormones are some of the strongest body chemicals. As a woman, I was well aware of the regular monthly variations in my own breasts that came with the hormonal changes of my menstrual cycle. My thought process was now moving like a freight train. My mind turned to the even greater hormone fluctuations that occur with pregnancy. Breast cells are particularly sensitive early in life, prior to puberty. Maybe, I speculated, they are even more vulnerable prior to birth, soon after they are formed.

It suddenly became crystal clear to me where I should have been looking all these years. Perhaps we had never looked far enough back in a woman's life for factors that affected her risk of breast cancer. Then I asked myself whether a tiny baby girl's breasts in utero could be forever impacted by the estrogens, growth factors, and other hormones that were omnipresent in such large doses during pregnancy.

FOR MY FRIEND JANE, AND ALL THE PREGNANT "JANES" IN THE WORLD

I didn't yet have data to verify or even investigate my hunch (although I soon would). But I did have a constant reminder of how important my work might be, if it panned out. My dear friend Jane was pregnant three times during this time of discovery. She and her growing tummy constantly inspired my thoughts. What I would learn could impact the future health of her babies—especially if they were girls. As it turned out, all three were girls.

And, as time would tell, related research from around the world would impact the future health of all babies, boys and girls, as they grew into men and women.

From the moment Jane was thinking about starting a family, she had confided in me that she wanted to do everything possible—to the letter— to give her baby-to-be (as it would turn out, her *babies*-to-be) the best chance of being born healthy and growing up strong. As a health professional herself, she knew that her baby's well-being at birth was dependent on how nutritiously she ate, how much weight she gained, abstaining from smoking and alcohol, taking multivitamins, and using medications only as advised by her doctor.

But neither of us had ever dreamed that conditions in the womb might *also predict future risk of breast cancer—and, as it would turn out, other diseases.*

Yes, it wasn't just me searching for clues to the origins of disease. Other researchers were also trying to pick up a new trail in their pursuit of the cause of cardiovascular disease. Certainly, a lot more was known about what causes this disease (commonly called atherosclerosis or hardening of the arteries), but epidemiologists always look for more.

Soon our research group at Harvard University and at least five other research teams around the world were deeply entrenched in this new area of study, exploring how a baby's environment in the womb can affect his or her well-being decades later. We thought not just of our pregnant friends but also of all the pregnant women in the world who would do anything to have a baby who was healthy at birth—and who also had the best chances of good health *throughout childhood, adolescence, and adulthood.*

SCIENCE UNDER THE SPOTLIGHT

Because conditions in the womb seem to affect future health, this novel research field is called fetal (or perinatal) origins of chronic disease. As I detail for you in Chapter One, the concept of fetal origins is not entirely new. It's just that recent advances have brought it to the public's attention. Some of the first evidence came from our grim observations of the children of Dutch women who were starved while pregnant during World War II (you'll read more about this in Chapter One). More recently, a British epidemiologist by the name of David Barker greatly advanced the concept with a flurry of research in the cardiovascular field that began in the 1980s. Today, with compelling new research results being touted both in scientific symposia *and* on the network news, one thing is clear: Our notions of the origins of adult health are undergoing nothing short of a revolution.

WHAT OUR RESEARCH MEANS FOR MOMS-TO-BE

Health professionals, including me, are now beginning to appreciate the far-reaching significance of the way a woman takes care of herself during pregnancy. Until recently, until this research started spilling forth such exciting results, we used to think that the most a woman could do by practicing sound nutrition was influence the health of her child at birth. *Now, we know that she—you—may be able to influence a baby's health at birth and long into adult life.*

I'm particularly excited by the fact that nutrition, even before birth, has turned out to be so important to long-term health. All my life my mom has been a great advocate of healthy eating. In fact, she was the person who first sparked my interest in nutrition; most of what I know about a healthy diet I learned from her. However, we never dreamed that nutrition during pregnancy could have such far-reaching ramifications!

That's why I wrote this book. Our findings are so important that it is time to share them with all of you who are pregnant or thinking of becoming pregnant. I want to help you give your child the best possible chance of being born healthy and living a long, robust life. Remember, though, we are only at the beginning of this revolutionary field of research and we have much to learn. But we did not want to wait for years until we had more scientific data before passing this important information on to you. Therefore, our recommendations and diet are based on the best research we have to date, combined with expert advice on good nutrition during pregnancy.

No matter where you are in your pregnancy, or even if you have already had your child—or you are looking back into *your own* birth history—there is every reason in the world to know about the fetal origins of chronic disease. Knowing about the factors being studied, including birth weight, head size, and birth length, can help you understand what potential health problems you (or your child) might be at risk for. Knowing what risks are accelerated, a person can try to counter them by living a defensive lifestyle and plan appropriate screening tests from an early age.

What you should know and keep in mind, also, is that the fetal origins concept does not outstrip everything else in importance when it comes to your child's adult health. You will appreciate, as you read this book, that neither conditions in the womb nor genetics, influential as they are, set our disease risk in stone. In other words, a person's whole life course, environment, and, in particular, lifestyle, are still of great importance in determining disease risk. This is why the emphasis on not smoking, keeping alcohol intake to safe levels, exercising regularly, and maintaining a healthy body weight is as strong as ever.

However, if you are pregnant now, or planning to have a child, you have a unique opportunity to put the breakthroughs of fetal origins of disease research into practice.

FROM THIS DAY FORWARD: EVERY DAY COUNTS!

I must emphasize again—more strongly, in fact—that you shouldn't worry if you are already pregnant that this information has escaped you so far. *No matter where you are in your pregnancy (or in the planning stages), what you do from this day forward can still favorably impact your child's future health profile.*

Indeed, there is so much to do and so much to worry about as you plan or go through your pregnancy. Do you need something else to make you crazy? Absolutely not. That's not the purpose of this book. While its purpose is to inform and help you, *just as importantly,* it's meant to soothe your fears, to give you hope. *The Gift of Health* is designed to simplify your life.

FROM THE SCIENCE TO THE DIET: USING *The Gift of Health*

As you peruse this book, you'll immediately see that it does more—*far more*—than describe the new research. It uses our breakthrough data on the fetal origins of chronic disease as a springboard for a surprisingly easy to follow, incredibly individualized diet and lifestyle plan any pregnant woman can implement to ensure the health of her child. I assure you, *The Gift of Health* is so complete that it's certain to be the only nutrition guide you'll ever put to use during your pregnancy. The following is a brief chapter-by-chapter description, so you'll see what I mean:

Chapter One provides an overview of the great and recent advances research has made in our understanding of the fetal origins of chronic disease. In Chapter Two, I explain in detail how the nutrition of a mom-to-be may affect her baby and can minimize his or her future risk of certain diseases.

In Chapter Three, "Goals, Objectives, and Calories . . . Calories . . . Calories: The Optimal Pregnancy Diet," you'll learn about the three major goals of eating and nutrition during pregnancy. In a nutshell, they are: (1) to prevent undernutrition during the first and third trimesters, (2) to prevent overnutrition in the second and third trimesters, and (3) to maximize the "notable nutrients" throughout pregnancy. These are the vitamins and minerals that my girlfriend Jane and I talked about so long ago (her oldest daughter is now 8!), those nutrients such as protein, vitamin B_6, calcium, folic acid, iron, and zinc that are especially important to fetal growth and development. At the same time, though, I'll be teaching you about every nutrient known to woman and how much you need throughout each trimester of pregnancy (including the "prepregnancy trimester," or those quintessential 3 months in training before you become pregnant.)

Chapter Three also gives you the lowdown on desired weight and calorie intake during pregnancy. In the section entitled "Calorie Madness," you'll see that our eating plan is different from all the rest. Knowing that no two expectant women are the same in their initial weights at conception or in their metabolic rates, I know that no one calorie intake level can meet the needs of all pregnant women. That's why you'll find a range of calorie levels. I'll guide you in your decision of which calorie level to begin at and in how to vary that calorie level as needed. For example, you may need to adjust your calorie intake up or down, depending on your individual rate of weight gain.

Chapter Four is one of the most consequential chapters in the book. It contains the "Don't Miss It" overview of the *Gift of Health* optimal pregnancy diet plan and can be considered a road map to the next four chapters. Each of Chapters Five through Eight is devoted to a trimester of pregnancy, preceded by one chapter for the vital few months before pregnancy, and each follows exactly the same format for ease of use. Following are some highlights from these chapters.

Chapter Five, "The Prepregnancy Optimal Diet": A prepregnancy diet? I must be kidding, right? This section is designed to help women get their bodies in shape, so to speak, for pregnancy. Consider this a training period prior to pregnancy, sort of like getting ready to run a big race. When a woman has the chance to prepare for pregnancy, she can ensure that all her cells are supernourished. This provides insurance that her body has optimal nutritional stores, including vitamins and minerals, at the time of conception and during the first crucial weeks of pregnancy. At this time, mothers may not yet know whether they are pregnant, and the fetus is particularly vulnerable to the effects of malnutrition. A range of three calorie levels is provided to allow women to either maintain their optimal weight (1,900 calories), lose weight slowly if they weigh more than 10% of their ideal weight (1,600 calories), and gain weight if they weigh less than 90% of their ideal weight (2,200 calories).

Of course, this is an ideal situation. Although I wholeheartedly recommend following these guidelines if you are planning a baby, I certainly do realize that pregnancies are often, shall I say, unexpected. Or, planned or not, you may get your hands on this book only later in your pregnancy. If this is the case, please don't fret. Simply jump in at whatever stage your pregnancy is at, remembering, as I said earlier, that what you do from this day forward will still have a positive effect on your child's future health.

Chapter Six, "The First-Trimester Optimal Diet" (weeks 1–13), has a primary goal of optimal nutrient intake combined with a weight gain of 3 to 6 pounds. Even this small amount of weight gain can seem like an insurmountable problem for some women who are extremely nauseated throughout this time. Thus, the meals plans focus on foods that are best tolerated when feeling nauseated while still providing 100% of the nutrients needed during this critical period of fetal development and placental growth. Here, I provide two calorie levels: 1,900 and 2,200.

Chapter Seven, "The Second-Trimester Optimal Diet" (weeks 14–26), covers a time when many women feel their best and have a very healthy appetite. It is also the time when cravings for high-calorie/high-fat foods commonly occur. Consequently, the second trimester is the time when excess weight gain is most likely to be a problem. We'll show you how to eat well during this trimester, giving you plenty of delicious yet nutritious escape hatches. (Try our too-good-to-be-true Banana Split, Banana Chocolate Chip Muffins, or Orange Cream Fruit Tarts to satisfy insurmountable cravings.) Our motto is that no food is off limits—we just help you plan for it in healthy amounts.

The Third-Trimester Optimal Diet (weeks 27 to 40), in Chapter Eight, emphasizes nutrient-dense foods and six small meals daily, rather than the three larger meals and three snacks eaten during the previous trimesters. This enables mothers to consume the amount of nutrients required to feed their rapidly growing babies despite feelings of fullness.

I have devoted Chapter Nine to women with diabetes and gestational diabetes. Exposing the fetus to high levels of glucose increases the risk of the baby developing diabetes as an adult. If the baby is a girl who goes on to develop gestational diabetes while pregnant, she may pass the disease down to a third generation. Thus, controlling blood glucose levels is more important during pregnancy than at any other time. This chapter not only provides general guidelines but also discusses modifications to the meal plans given in the previous chapters.

Chapter Ten showcases our mouthwatering recipes. I've teamed up with registered dietitian and culinary wizard Kristine Napier, MPH, RD,

LD, to translate theory into food—what to put on your plate at each meal and even between meals.

You'll love the fabulously delicious and easy-to-follow menu plans and accompanying recipes developed by Kristine just for you. They're specific to your appetite as it changes trimester by trimester. The recipes included in this chapter correspond to those given in the menu plans for each trimester (Chapters Five through Eight). One of the best aspects of our menu system? Within each trimester's meal plan, every breakfast is interchangeable with every other breakfast; the same is true of the lunches and the dinners. For you, that means mixing and matching these meals in countless ways to create enough menu plans for your whole pregnancy. We'll also show you how simple it is to create your own menus if you want to venture out from those we provide (and we encourage you to do so!).

Here's an extra bonus within our 103 recipes: You'll find plenty that are ideal for a romantic dinner with your partner or for feeding the whole family. And we've thought of those pregnancy cravings, building in Cheesy Spinach Pizza, Chocolate Fudge Brownies and The Best Hamburger. We guarantee you'll use these recipes again and again, both during your pregnancy and in the years that follow.

In the last chapter, Chapter Eleven, I put all of the information I've provided throughout the book into a healthy perspective. The most important advice I want to leave you with: No one should ever blame Mom for all her ills. Although the new science of fetal origins of disease may position us on a new frontier, we still have many roads to travel before we reach our final destination. What this means to you is that I am not promising a magic bullet—at least not yet. And don't fear that sidestepping some of my advice will totally derail the health of your baby. Lifestyle and genetics, as I have mentioned, still play a strong role (although less than was once believed) in adult illness and disease. Conditions in the womb may, however, influence our health for life. And exceptional nutrition during the three trimesters of pregnancy, and the preceding months, is one path that will help to keep you and your baby moving in the right direction.

I am finally realizing my wish to help women fight diseases such as breast cancer and may be making some headway in understanding who should be more vigilant when it comes to breast cancer screening. I had never dared to dream that my research could have such far-reaching ramifications. At the same time, I'm thrilled to share the excitement of so many of my colleagues who are uncovering the link between other common adult diseases and conditions in the womb. In its broadest sense, all this wondrous research really does one very simple thing: It enables pregnant women to learn how to care for themselves in the best way possible, which will help ensure that they have healthy babies, and that these babies have the greatest chance of living a long, healthy life.

Here's to a happy, healthy, and easy pregnancy!

Dr. Karin B. Michels

CHAPTER ONE

———————————————— 🍎 ————————————————

The Science

Eating for Your Child's Future

"What do you want? A boy? Or a girl?"

If you're expecting, or are even thinking about getting pregnant, no doubt you've heard that question a thousand times by now. You may be secretly hoping for either a little son or daughter, but like most expectant mothers, you have an even more important wish: "I just want a healthy baby." Certainly, this overriding concern will be uppermost in your mind in the delivery room until the doctor or midwife proclaims, "The baby is perfect!"

Now, I want you to take this lovely scenario one giant step further. As if in a time machine, think about your baby's health years later, *when he or she is an adult.* A new branch of science—the basis of this book—provides evidence that how you take care of yourself during pregnancy can do much more than give your unborn child a great start in life. You can also help reduce his or her risk of several common and serious diseases that strike in adulthood, ensuring the health of the adult your baby will eventually become.

MARGARET'S STORY

Forty-nine-year-old Margaret exercises regularly, eats a low-fat diet, maintains a trim body weight, and doesn't smoke. Still, she has already had a double bypass because of coronary artery disease (hardening of the arteries that supply blood to the heart) that was causing chest pain and shortness of breath. On top of that, she was recently diagnosed with

adult-onset diabetes. Margaret always thought that these health problems happened only to overweight couch potatoes who ate large amounts
of French fries and cheesecake. Trying to understand the source of her
maladies, Margaret's doctor asked if she had a family history of these illnesses, but searching through the family tree revealed no links.

Startling new research that I alluded to above may provide a clue about
the genesis of Margaret's health woes. At least part of the explanation may
trace much further back than we've ever thought possible—to the days
before her birth, to Margaret's time in her mother's womb.

THE CONCEPT

Scientists call this revolutionary new field of study the fetal origins of
chronic disease. *Fetal origins* refers simply to the growing realization that
some adult conditions, such as heart disease and breast cancer, may be
impacted by conditions during pregnancy. It is meant to convey how life
in the womb impacts not only the baby that is born but also the adult he
or she will one day become. The fetal environment is shaped by the nutrients and the hormones that flow from mother to baby. In turn, these are
partially influenced by a mom's diet, how much weight she gains, and the
pattern in which she gains weight.

Fetal origins research focuses on the long-lasting effects of either positive or negative conditions at a sensitive or critical period of development
of the baby's organs, tissue, and other body systems while in the womb.
Examples of sensitive periods of development are when heart tissue dif-
ferentiates into the four heart chambers or when the number of fat cells
is decided. Two quintessential examples of negative conditions are undernutrition and overnutrition. Others can occur when the mother takes
drugs, smokes, or drinks alcohol.

The fetal environment is critical to the health of the developing baby
and the adult she or he will become because budding tissues are pliable,
which means they can easily be molded and reshaped. By design, fetal
tissues have to be pliable because they grow so rapidly and must differen-
tiate into so many different types of cells, from liver and kidney cells to
brain and muscle cells. To create a visual image of these happenings,
think of the elasticity of a balloon. Only because it is elastic or pliable can
it grow so fast and change when you blow air into it. In a very simplistic
sense, a developing fetus must be just as elastic to grow as rapidly as
nature intended. The elasticity that is so necessary also means that fetal

tissue can be affected—in both positive and negative ways—by the environment in which it is developing.

THE BIRTH OF AN IDEA

The concept of fetal origins of chronic disease, although revolutionary in that recent advances have finally brought it to the public's attention, is not entirely new. Let's take a look back in history.

Fetal origins was born of observations made in the mid-twentieth century. We learned important things about the effect of maternal nutrition on babies' future health from the tragedies of World War II. Autumn 1944 brought two huge problems to people in the western area of the Netherlands: a Nazi blockade of supplies and an early, hard winter. Together, they triggered a famine, which came to be called the Hunger Winter, or Dutch Famine.

Food became so scarce that people from the city fled to the countryside to scavenge for food and soon took to eating tulip bulbs. According to records kept during that time, the daily calorie intake in January 1945 dropped to a dangerously low 750, and soon after, most people were eating a mere 500 calories daily. (In comparison, nutritionists know that most women, depending on their age, gender, and physical activity level, need 1,700 to 2,100 calories daily to maintain a healthy weight, and pregnant women require 1,900 to 2,200.)

By the time the Hunger Winter ended on May 5, 1945, it had taken the lives of 20,000 people. Some two decades later, the husband-and-wife research team of Mervyn Susser and Zena Stein found that it had also impacted the lives of those in the womb during the famine. Studying the people who had been conceived during or before the famine, Susser and Stein found many consequences of starvation conditions in the womb. Babies poorly nourished early in pregnancy, when the body organs are forming, had an increased risk of central nervous system birth defects, such as spina bifida, but paradoxically enough, also a substantially increased risk of being overweight as an adult. Continuing his parents' early research in the 1980s, Ezra Susser found that fetuses who were poorly nourished early on in pregnancy were also twice as likely to develop schizophrenia as fetuses who were well nourished.

Moving the Concept Forward in Expanding Research

As I mentioned in the Introduction, it was a British epidemiologist, David Barker, at the Medical Research Council Environmental Epidemiology Unit at the University of Southampton who greatly advanced the concept of fetal origins of disease. He also introduced the term *fetal programming* to explain his observations. Since 1986, Dr. Barker and his team have published over 200 scientific articles supporting his hypothesis that part of our risk of cardiovascular disease and diabetes in adulthood is "programmed" while we are in our mother's womb. (So pivotal were his findings that the concept of fetal programming as it pertains to cardiovascular disease is often called The Barker Hypothesis.) Other research teams, including mine, have enthusiastically joined in these exciting and critically important investigations of life in the womb and its effect on babies' future health risks.

Applying the results from this research to a woman's pregnancy—to your days in waiting—may give us the chance to prevent many cases of heart disease, diabetes, hypertension, obesity, mental illness, cancer, and other common diseases that have such a negative impact on so many people's lives. And we may be able to stop these diseases literally before they begin.

Nutrition: A Critical Prenatal Environment

The primary environment I'm discussing in this book is the nutrition mom provides to her developing child. But I'll also help you understand the role drugs and other lifestyle factors have in the process. In Chapter Eleven, I explain how exposures during the entire course of a person's life modify the effect the early events may have. Do also note that a mom's nutrition can impact the hormones her body produces and that these, in turn, can also affect the environment in the womb. We'll talk more about that in the next chapters.

As an aside, scientists know that the impact of early life course events doesn't stop at birth; it extends into early infancy. A famous example noted by researchers in this area is that of early twentieth-century Japanese soldiers and settlers taken to climates much hotter than they were accustomed to. Japanese physiologists noted that there was a wide variety of responses to the sweltering heat, and they soon discovered that the people who "took the heat better," or who cooled down faster, had more functioning sweat glands.

Further study revealed why some people have more functioning sweat glands than others. At birth, everyone has the same number of sweat glands, but none of them function. Conditions during the first 3 years determine, or "program," what proportion of those sweat glands become functional. As it turns out, babies growing up in warmer conditions during the first 3 years of life "program" more sweat glands to become functional than do infants raised in cooler conditions early in life and hence will be more comfortable living in a hot climate.

THE ROLE OF EPIDEMIOLOGY, OR WHERE MEDICINE MEETS MATH

As I detail in the next section of this chapter, researchers got an inkling about the far-reaching effects of life in the womb and the fetal origins of disease after noticing that adults with greater risks of cardiovascular disease, diabetes, and chronic bronchitis were more likely to have been born tiny.

Noticing that specific lifestyle or environmental or genetic factors are more common in people with certain health conditions is the basis of the science of epidemiology. It was the field of epidemiology that allowed scientists to make the associations that led to the development of the fetal origins hypothesis.

Epidemiology is my area of expertise. Epidemiologists are detectives trying to uncover the relation between risk factors and specific diseases. As epidemiologists, we study the characteristics of people who all suffer from a certain disease. For example, the critical knowledge that smoking is an important causal factor for lung cancer came after epidemiologists discovered that the majority of those afflicted were smokers.

Certainly, not all risk factor–disease relations have such a direct association. In fact, some relations that seem to offer a clue as to why diseases occur are subsequently found to be noncausal and the factor identified is only an innocent bystander to the association between a second factor and disease. For example, a study may reveal that people who get lung cancer are more likely to carry matches than people without lung cancer. We know today that carrying matches is only a marker for the true risk factor, smoking. But such observations are what ultimately allow epidemiologists to discover the clues to what causes disease—and that's the first step in finding effective means of preventing disease.

One of the ways epidemiologists find clues to the causes of disease is to map the geographical occurrence of the disease in question. Then, they superimpose on the map nondisease factors such as affluence (reflected in the gross national product, or GNP), living conditions, or dietary habits. When simultaneous pockets crop up—say, an infectious disease such as influenza is found to occur more frequently in areas of poverty—epidemiologists have a clue that they may be related; for example, that crowded living conditions and unsanitary quarters may play some role. Indeed, this is a well-known relation to experts on infectious disease.

Once clues are uncovered in one population, epidemiologists seek to find the same association in other groups of people. This is called replicating the data. If the data cannot be replicated, then the initial clues are more likely regarded as coincidental, or spurious, in epidemiologic terms.

Another key step in drawing a relation between an apparent risk factor and a disease is to account for other factors. This is called controlling for confounders. For example, when studying the link between smoking and heart disease, researchers have "to control for" or take into account the nutritional intake of smokers. This is because smokers often don't eat as well as nonsmokers, and poor nutrition can also increase the risk of heart disease.

Once epidemiologists collect all the data, they try to determine if one factor or a combination of factors increases the occurrence of a certain condition. Then, they calculate the difference in disease frequency between people with and without this factor. The next step is to apply statistical standards to decide if this difference is within the normal "plus or minus" category or if it is so different that it is unlikely to be due to chance and is thus called "statistically significant."

Here's an analogy: If you were making a quilt and were cutting out squares of fabric for the design by first tracing a pattern onto the fabric and then cutting out the squares, each one you cut would be slightly different from the next. A tiny bit of difference wouldn't matter—it would be within the normal give-and-take—but if one square was considerably off, it would be so different as to be noticeable. It would, in epidemiologic terms, be significantly different.

EARLY EVIDENCE FOR THE FETAL ORIGINS OF DISEASE: CORONARY HEART DISEASE

After the early leads from the Dutch Hunger Winter, scientists in England focused on the role of the fetal environment in the development of coronary heart disease (CHD), commonly known as atherosclerosis; it is the process by which the arteries that nourish the heart become clogged.

In 1984, Dr. David Barker was puzzling over maps of England detailing concentrated pockets of disease. One disease pattern he and his colleagues were studying was CHD. The team was simultaneously looking at maps detailing other factors, including a map showing pockets of neonatal mortality during the early 1900s.

The Barker epidemiology group's close scrutiny revealed a big surprise: The same areas that had a high incidence of contemporary CHD had a very high rate of neonatal mortality in the early 1900s. It had already been found that babies born smaller than expected—that is, with a very low birth weight—were more likely to die in the neonatal period. That same research showed that when there were pockets of neonatal mortality, those same geographical pockets also had a large number of babies born with very low birth weight who survived. Dr. Barker's stroke of genius was to ask the right question: Could it be that the babies who were born so small but survived anyway were the ones who had a higher chance of heart disease as adults?

This idea was intriguing but seemed counterintuitive. Conventional wisdom held that the two phenomena should be unrelated. After all, neonatal mortality is more likely to occur in poverty-stricken populations, because neonatal care is often lacking, as is good nutrition for the mom and therefore for the developing baby.

In contrast, heart experts—then, as today—think of cardiovascular disease as the consequence of excesses: too much food, too many calories, too much dietary fat, too many excess pounds, and too little physical activity. *These adult lifestyle factors remain significant contributors to CHD.* But Dr. Barker's discoveries taught us that adult excesses don't explain the whole picture.

Trying to "connect the dots" between the neonatal mortality data and adult heart disease, Dr. Barker set out on a mission to find data that might give clues to the association. If there was an answer, it would lie in birth records dating from the early 1900s.

The problem was tracking down such old files. To facilitate the search, he and his team enlisted the help of a University of Oxford historian. His detective work was a fascinating part of the story. Birth records turned up in archives, lofts, sheds, garages, boiler rooms, and flooded basements. The most complete—and helpful—records turned up in Hertfordshire, a shire (similar to a county in the United States) in the south of England. A health official known as the "lady inspector of midwives" had kept meticulous records on every baby born from 1911 onwards in that shire.*

The Barker epidemiology team delved into the records describing the births of approximately 16,000 men and women from 1911 to 1930, matching them with death certificates, in particular, death certificates that stated cardiovascular disease. It didn't take the researchers long to make the connection. They found that Dr. Barker's initial, seemingly odd hypothesis about low birth weight and adult risk of heart disease had struck a bull's-eye.

According to these data, men and women who weighed 5.5 pounds at birth or less had almost double the chance of dying of cardiovascular disease (both coronary artery disease and stroke) than those with a birth weight of more than 9.5 pounds. The researchers delved deeper into the issue of low birth weight: Was it low because the baby was born too early (in which case a lower birth weight is expected), or was it low because the baby didn't grow properly in utero but went full term? In the latter case, conditions in the womb are not optimal; for instance, a mom might not have gotten proper nutrition. After investigating this question, the researchers found that in the majority of cases, low birth weight was associated with an increased incidence of cardiovascular disease later in life for babies who were born full term but who didn't grow properly in utero. Incidentally, the association remained even after the investigators accounted for socioeconomic differences and other adult life risk factors for cardiovascular disease.

Just another note about how researchers regard low birth weights. In addition to asking the question about whether or not the baby was of low birth weight because of being born too early or because of suboptimal growing conditions in the womb, researchers compare birth weight to birth length and head circumference. The three factors should correspond to each other. When a baby is thin for his or her length and/or has a head that is disproportionately large, he or she probably didn't have the

*Recording of birth weight and infant health was maintained until 1945 in Hertfordshire.

benefit of optimal growing conditions. The most common culprit: Mom's poor nutrition.

RESEARCH ON FETAL ORIGINS AND HEART DISEASE CONTINUES

Today, the strongest evidence about the fetal origins of disease comes from its link to cardiovascular disease.

Such a link is apparent in India, where the average birth weight is below 6 pounds (2.7 kilograms), much lower than the norm of 7.1 to 8.5 pounds (3.2–3.9 kilograms) for girls and 7.0 to 8.4 pounds (3.2–3.8 kilograms) for boys in developed countries. Dr. Barker's research team found this link after scrutinizing the birth records of 517 men and women born during the period between 1934 and 1953 in one hospital in south India and then looking at their current health records. The researchers discovered almost a fourfold increase in the rate of CHD for those born very small: The prevalence of CHD was 15% in those who weighed 5.5 pounds (2.5 kilograms) or less at birth, in contrast to 4% in the group who weighed 7.0 pounds (3.2 kilograms) or more. Just as with the group of people born in Hertfordshire, England, the association became even stronger when researchers separated out those babies who had low birth weight at full term, due to adverse conditions in the womb, from those who had low birth weight just because they were born too early.

Further analysis uncovered yet another association: Those with the highest rates of heart disease were more likely to have been born to mothers who were considered too thin during pregnancy. This discovery about low maternal weight provided more important evidence that poor fetal growth as a consequence of undernutrition during pregnancy may lead to coronary artery disease.

My Harvard colleagues, led by Dr. Janet Rich-Edwards, have also studied birth weight and the incidence of heart disease, analyzing both the birth weight and adult health information of 70,797 women from a large and very well known study population, the Nurses' Health Study.

To give greater credence to any associations that might surface, my Harvard colleagues used very stringent criteria for heart disease. In addition, they tightened their study even further by controlling for, or taking into account, several factors that are known or suspected to increase heart disease risk, such as adult body weight, high blood pressure, diabetes, and dietary factors. In research, we use the term *control for* to mean that we have taken into account extenuating circumstances that could distort the results.

The results confirmed those of earlier studies: the lower the birth weight, the greater the risk of heart disease. Women with a birth weight of 5.5 pounds or less (2.5 kilograms or less) had a 23% greater risk of heart disease compared with women born weighing more than 5.5 pounds. As the August 16, 1997, issue of the prestigious *British Medical Journal* reported, their study provided "strong evidence of an association between birth weight and adult coronary heart disease and stroke."

PRENATAL CONDITIONS AND HYPERTENSION

According to the American Heart Association, one in four Americans has hypertension, or high blood pressure. Worse than having high blood pressure is lack of knowledge about it: An alarming one third of affected people don't know their blood pressure hovers at a dangerously elevated level.

In the vast majority of people with hypertension, there is no apparent cause. Hypertension without an identifiable cause is called "essential hypertension." Now, researchers of early life think that fetal conditions in the womb may offer at least a partial explanation of why essential hypertension occurs.

One of the first findings Dr. Barker made after examining health records from the Hertfordshire residents was that low birth weight raised the risk of suffering hypertension as an adult. Subsequent studies of people in different parts of England confirmed that low birth weight upped the incidence of adult hypertension.

In these next studies, researchers asked another question: Was the hypertension found in infants who had been born full term but small for their age, or in babies who had a low birth weight because they were born prematurely? Obviously, conditions in the womb would have been different in the two groups. The answer was clear: The hypertension was found in babies born at term but smaller than normal, babies who had received less nutrition than they needed before birth. This further strengthened the relation between low birth weight and adult hypertension.

To date, in Europe alone, the health records of over 8,000 adults have been compared to their birth weights. The results have been reported in more than 40 articles in the medical literature. Consistently, these studies have confirmed that low birth weight raises the risk of suffering hypertension as an adult.

In the United States, the birth weight of nearly 185,000 people has been related to their frequency of developing hypertension. My Harvard colleagues who analyzed data from the two Nurses' Health Studies and the male equivalent, the Health Professionals' Follow-Up Study, investigated the low birth weight–adult hypertension association in over 160,000 women and nearly 23,000 men. As do the European studies, these U.S. studies provide evidence that birth weight predicts adult risk of hypertension.

PRENATAL CONDITIONS AND ADULT WEIGHT PROBLEMS

While we've learned from the observations about birth weight and heart disease that it's not good to be born too small, the next lesson is that tipping the scales in the other direction at birth is not advantageous, either. I guess you'd say that striving for a happy medium—a healthy average birth weight—is best of all.

A weight problem in adult life was one of the first conditions found to be related to life in the womb. This revelation came from the tragedy of World War II you read about earlier in this chapter, the Nazis' attempt to starve the people of western Holland. Babies who were conceived during the famine—and therefore were undernourished during their first trimester—were surprisingly far more likely to become overweight as adults.

The next wave of research on fetal life and adult weight produced a new, and seemingly contradictory, revelation: Being too well fed in the womb and being born much heavier than the norm also significantly increases the risk of adult weight problems. Colleagues of mine at Harvard University, led by Gary C. Curhan, MD, used the three large studies mentioned above to search for a connection between birth weight and becoming overweight as an adult.

Women, Their Birth Weight, and Their Risk of Adult Weight Problems

One study population was a group of women from the Nurses' Health Study mentioned above in the heart disease discussion. The researchers compared the women's birth weight with their body mass index, or BMI, a measure that tells whether a person is underweight, normal weight, or overweight. (We'll talk more about BMI in Chapter Three.) Compared

with women who weighed between 7.1 and 8.5 pounds at birth, the optimal birth weight for females, those born with a birth weight greater than
10 pounds had a 62% greater chance of becoming overweight. Women
born with a weight between 8.6 and 10 pounds still had a 19% increased
risk of becoming overweight.*

Men, Their Birth Weight, and Adult Obesity Risk

Similar results for men emerged from our large study of nearly 52,000
male health-care professionals. Compared with men born in the optimal
weight range (7.0 to 8.4 pounds), those born at 10 pounds or greater had
more than a 200% increased risk of being overweight.

How can starvation conditions early in pregnancy produce the same
consequence as overabundance in the last trimester? This has to do with
two different critical or sensitive periods of development. Refer to
Chapter Three, pages 58 and 59, for a complete explanation of this seemingly paradoxical situation.

Determinants of Birth Weight

**Like other conditions influenced by the environment in the womb,
birth weight is determined by a complex mix of factors. Scientists
have found that high birth weight may be related to:**

- **Maternal diabetes mellitus (blood sugar abnormalities)**
- **High maternal prepregnancy weight**
- **Excessive maternal weight gain during pregnancy**
- **Prolonged gestation**
- **High maternal levels of estrogens and/or growth hormones**

See Chapter Two for more information on these factors.

---

*Women with a birth weight of less than 5 pounds were also somewhat more likely to
become overweight. Birth weight and adult weight seem to be connected by a U-shaped
curve: being at either extreme end of the distribution is undesirable.

PRENATAL CONDITIONS AND BODY SHAPE: APPLES VERSUS PEARS

For adults (and even children and adolescents), excess weight alone is bad enough in terms of increasing the risk of diseases such as heart disease, diabetes, and hypertension. But continued study of weight problems has taught us that *where* people store their surplus pounds may be just as important as how much extra weight they gain.

To be more specific, we now know that carrying excess weight around the waist more rapidly increases the risk of diabetes and heart disease. In medical terms, people who carry excess weight around the waist are said to have "abdominal obesity." More commonly, this is called having an apple shape. On the other hand, people who carry their excess weight below the belt, on their hips and upper thighs (called a pear shape) don't tend to have such an elevated risk of the diseases noted.

A child with a low birth weight is more likely to be apple-shaped as an adult. We first learned this from the men in Hertfordshire, England. Three other studies, (one of 30-year-old Mexican and non-Hispanic Americans, one of English teenage girls, and a third of children aged 7 to 12 years in Philadelphia) confirmed this relation between low birth weight and the chance of being apple-shaped.

LIFE IN THE WOMB AND DIABETES MELLITUS

An estimated 14 million to 15 million Americans have type 2 diabetes mellitus (also called adult-onset diabetes), the most common type of diabetes or blood sugar abnormality. With this disease, it's not just that blood sugars run too high. Today, the complications of diabetes, such as heart disease, kidney damage, nerve damage, and cancer, make type 2 diabetes the seventh leading cause of death in the United States. Alarmingly, one third of people with type 2 diabetes don't know their blood sugars are raging out of control and possibly damaging their body systems.

Although being overweight and leading a sedentary lifestyle put a person at increased risk of this type of diabetes, not everyone who develops it is obese. The environment in the womb may be one factor that influences a person's risk of diabetes mellitus, as we first learned from the people in Hertfordshire. In a group of 370 men, the risk of diabetes was increased nearly sevenfold in those born very small, which means they had low weight gain while in the womb.

My Harvard colleagues also queried our databases for such an association, confirming these earlier results. The Nurses' Health Study uncovered a 83% increased risk of diabetes in women born weighing under
5 pounds, compared with those born in the normal range of 7.1 to 8.5
pounds, and a 76% increased risk for women born weighing between
5 and 5.5 pounds. The risk was still slightly elevated—at 23%—in women
born between 5.6 and 7.0 pounds. To clarify the genesis of their results,
the researchers controlled for (or took into account) all the other things
that may increase the risk for diabetes, including whether or not the
women studied were overweight or had a family history of diabetes, the
women's ethnicity, and their adult lifestyle factors.

CONDITIONS IN THE WOMB AND BREAST CANCER RISK

Now, on to my area of research—life in the womb and breast cancer. As I
described to you in the Introduction when I told you how I embarked on
this line of research, the breast is very vulnerable to hormones, growth
factors, and other substances that can act as carcinogens (substances that
may cause cancer). For reasons I'll explain in Chapter Two, this is especially true when a tiny baby girl is in the womb.

Before I started my research on prenatal influences on breast cancer, I
had learned a lot from my colleagues who work on animal models and
who described how vulnerable the breast tissue of a young female rat is in
the first days of life. I also received a huge impetus from my epidemiology
pal and dear friend from Sweden, Dr. Anders Ekbom. Dr. Ekbom, a sur-
geon and epidemiologist, was similarly obsessed with unveiling the
causes of breast cancer. He is a very gifted scientist, full of innovative
ideas and new concepts regarding why things are the way they are and
which avenues we should pursue in our quest for the causes of cancer.
Anders Ekbom has done some pioneering work in Sweden: He was fortunate to have some data on women's health during pregnancy and on their
offsprings' health status. He found that women who suffered from a special condition called preeclampsia during pregnancy were much less
likely to have daughters who developed breast cancer as adults. The main
symptoms of preeclampsia are protein in the urine and high blood pressure during pregnancy. Dr. Ekbom was puzzled by this startling observation, but he is very clever, and he was aware of one important fact:
Women who experience preeclampsia generally have lower pregnancy

estrogen levels. Could it be that these pregnancy estrogen levels played a role in the female baby's future breast cancer risk?

Pregnancy estrogen levels also influence birth weight. Although I realized this could be a factor in future breast cancer risk, it was not my only consideration as I approached the question of whether this disease was influenced by conditions prior to birth. I wanted to know about everything that happened during the mother's pregnancy: what she ate, how much she weighed, how much weight she gained, whether she drank coffee or alcohol, whether she smoked, whether she experienced nausea, whether she took prescription drugs, how much the baby weighed at birth, whether the baby was born prematurely or carried to term, whether the baby was breast-fed or bottle-fed, and so on. I was lucky to have the opportunity to tag on to two very large studies of women that were (and still are) going on at Harvard University: the previously mentioned Nurses' Health Study and its younger equivalent, the Nurses' Health Study II. I was equally fortunate to get a research grant to pursue my plans. We already knew a lot about these nurses, including their health status and whether they had breast cancer, but we needed to find out about their mothers! So I mailed questionnaires to the nurses' mothers, asking them about everything they did and experienced during their pregnancy with their nurse daughter, and I named the study the Nurses' Mothers' Study.

Naturally, it took some time to collect all the relevant data and have it entered into our computer system, but finally, the day arrived when I could begin my analyses. It was a rainy Monday morning in February 1995 in Boston, and I was sitting in my office in the Department of Epidemiology at the Harvard School of Public Health. I had skimmed through the data during the previous week and I had not noticed anything in particular. Then, that morning, I decided to focus on the analysis of birth weight. I related the birth weight of the nurses, as reported to us by their mothers, to the frequency of breast cancer among the nurses. When the computer spilled out the results, I could not believe my eyes! I looked at the printout again and again. The data staring at me told me that women weighing 5.5 pounds (2.5 kg) or less at birth had half the risk of breast cancer than women who weighed 8.8 pounds (4 kg) or more when they were born. But there was another thing about my data that struck me almost more. It is very rare in epidemiology that we see a clear association between a factor and a disease across all levels of that factor. The relation between birth weight and breast cancer risk was a straight line: the higher the birth weight, the higher the frequency of breast cancer among the women I was studying. I had never seen anything like this in my career as an epidemiologist. I was so excited I had to share the news! It just so happened that my friend, Anders Ekbom, was visiting the department that day. I rushed up the stairs and ran into him in the hall: "Anders, Anders, you won't believe this—it's a straight line!" Of course, Dr. Ekbom did not know what I was referring to, but when I showed him my data, he smiled. He was not really surprised. We shared the news with Dr. Dimitrios Trichopoulos, another distinguished breast cancer epidemiologist and supporter of the theory that prenatal factors might influence breast cancer risk. He looked at my computer printout and just nodded his head. Our hypothesis was confirmed.

We succeeded in publishing our findings in the prestigious medical journal *The Lancet*, which resulted in a great deal of international attention for our research. But, of course, we have not stopped at birth weight. Our quest continues to identify more factors that influence the unborn child's risk of cancer.

PRENATAL LIFE AND PROSTATE CANCER

My Swedish research colleagues, led by Dr. Anders Ekbom, studied the cancer incidence of a group of 366 men born in 1913 in Gothenburg, Sweden. The men were enrolled in the study and their birth weight was known from midwife records. The medical team tracked them for the development of prostate cancer. During 30 years of observation, 21 of the 366 men developed prostate cancer.

The research team then divided the men into birth weight categories and checked to see if there was any difference in the occurrence of prostate cancer by birth weight category. Indeed there was. Men born in the highest one fourth of the birth weight range, or above 8.7 pounds, were five times more likely to develop prostate cancer as an adult than were men in the lower three quarters of birth weight range (below 8.7 pounds).

CONDITIONS IN THE WOMB AND TESTICULAR CANCER

The risk of developing testicular cancer also seems related to birth weight. Some early research suggested that the hormonal milieu during gestation could influence the later risk of developing testicular cancer. This is what led Dr. Ekbom and my other Swedish colleagues to delve further into how life in the womb might impact the future risk of testicular cancer.

They studied 232 men with invasive testicular cancer, comparing them with 904 men of similar age and socioeconomic status. They analyzed the research in even greater detail: They separated the men with testicular cancer into the two main types of this cancer, seminoma and nonseminoma cancer. The testes contains different types of tissue, one of which includes the tubules that transfer semen. Tumors that affect this type of tissue are called seminomas, whereas those that affect the other tissue in the testes are called nonseminomas.

When both types of tumors were analyzed together, the researchers found that those men with either a low or a high birth weight had an increased risk of testicular cancer in adult life. Those men born at a birth weight below 5.5 pounds had a risk about 2.5 times that of men born at an average birth weight, whereas men born heavier than the average, with a birth weight greater than or equal to 8.8 pounds, had a risk that was increased about 1.5 times. When the research team divided the men into two groups on the basis of their type of tumor, they found that the low birth weight was more likely to be associated with nonseminoma tumors. On the other hand, it was a heavier placenta (which is weighed after a baby is delivered) rather than birth weight that was far more likely to be associated with seminoma tumors (you'll read more about the relevance of placental weight in Chapter Two).

PRENATAL LIFE AND CHILDHOOD CANCERS

Cancer is a little-understood disease, causing much fear—especially when it occurs in children. Epidemiologists from around the world have found evidence that prenatal factors, or life in the womb, may impact the risk of certain childhood cancers.

Cancer researchers from the Fred Hutchinson Cancer Research Center in Seattle conducted one of the first studies that documented a tendency for children with higher birth weight to have a higher risk of cancer during childhood. They found that among children diagnosed with cancer during the first several years of life, there was an increased proportion with a high birth weight, or a birth weight over 8.8 pounds. The risk was most pronounced for children under age 2 years, and was virtually absent after age 4.

Perhaps the most common malignancy, or cancer, in children is leukemia—in particular, a type of leukemia called acute lymphatic leukemia. Previous research found that certain genetic disorders, including Down syndrome, as well as being an identical twin increases the risk of developing acute lymphatic leukemia. Because this type of cancer peaks in occurrence at 2 to 4 years of age, researchers have long speculated that prenatal factors play a role in its cause.

Dr. Ekbom's team in Sweden studied 613 children with acute lymphatic leukemia, and compared them with over 3,000 children of similar age and with similar other characteristics. They found that several prenatal factors were associated with an increased risk. One was birth weight: They found that babies weighing more than 9.9 pounds at birth had a 70% increased risk of developing this type of leukemia as very young children. Another prenatal factor that increased the risk of acute lymphatic leukemia was maternal hypertension, which accelerated the risk by 40%.

A Danish team of researchers studied children with two other types of leukemia, acute lymphoblastic leukemia (ALL) and acute myeloid leukemia (AML) to try to identify risk factors. As did the Swedish group that studied acute lymphatic leukemia, the Danish researchers found that higher birth weight increased the risk of these two other forms of leukemia. For both subtypes of leukemia, they found that increasing birth weight over the average of 7.7 pounds increased the risk. The increased risk for ALL was about 1.5 times, whereas for AML, the risk was over twice as much.

Brain cancer is the second most frequent type of cancer in children under the age of 14 in the United States. Researchers from the Johns Hopkins School of Hygiene and Public Health in Maryland and the National Cancer Institute delved into the possible risk factors for brain tumors in children. They found that children with brain tumors (as well as children with other cancers) were more likely to have been born with higher birth weights. Specifically, they found that children weighing more than 8.0 pounds at birth had 2.6 times the risk of developing a brain tumor.*

PRENATAL LIFE AND ASTHMA

Researchers from four different corners of the globe—Australia, Germany, Great Britain, and the United States—have studied how life in the womb influences the development of childhood asthma.

---

*Several other research groups have confirmed these observations.

Australian researchers, led by Dr. William H. Kitchen, studied nearly 600 children born between 1977 and 1982, dividing them into three birth weight groups. One group consisted of infants born at very low birth weight, less than 2.2 pounds. Another group was composed of infants who weighed between 2.2 and 5.5 pounds. The last group was composed of 60 children weighing more than 5.5 pounds at birth. The children were examined at the age of 8 years for the presence of asthma symptoms, which included wheezing; they also underwent pulmonary (lung) function tests that revealed the presence of asthma. These researchers found no compelling evidence that respiratory health at 8 years of age was related to perinatal events.

German researchers, however, did find an association. Their research, of 1,812 children, found that a lower birth weight was associated with childhood risk of having asthma: Children with a birth weight under 5.5 pounds were two times more likely to suffer from asthma symptoms. This team of researchers also found evidence that a woman smoking during pregnancy increased the risk of her child suffering from asthma symptoms during childhood.

Similarly, the British research team, led by Dr. S. Lewis of the City University of London, found that low birth weight and maternal smoking increased the risk that a child would suffer asthma. A birth weight less than 5.5 pounds increased the risk by 26%. Babies born to mothers who smoked 15 or more cigarettes during pregnancy had a 39% increased risk of developing asthma. Interestingly, these risk percentages were higher in babies who were boys. Low birth weight and maternal smoking appear to operate independently from each other, but each seems to be related to asthma-associated wheezing by the time children are 5 years old. The researchers also found that asthma associated with low birth weight or maternal smoking generally goes away by the teenage years, namely 16 years of age. Asthma persisting after age 16 is generally thought to be due to factors other than low birth weight or maternal smoking, such as low maternal age and high socioeconomic status. Researchers do not fully understand why high socioeconomic status increases the risk of asthma. They do believe that high socioeconomic status is simply a marker for something in the lifestyle that increases asthma risk. Research continues to try to sort this out.

A fourth research team came from the United States and was composed of medical experts from the U.S. Environmental Protection Agency and a multidisciplinary team from Harvard University and Harvard Medical School. They analyzed data from the Second National Health and Nutritional Examination Survey (NHANES II), which was conducted between February 1976 and February 1980. Included among the over 20,000–plus people in this study were 5,672 children aged 11 years and younger.

Among other factors, the researchers found that low birth weight (below 7.2 pounds) increased the risk of having childhood asthma by 40%. Like the British researchers, the American team found that the likelihood of getting asthma as a child was greater in boys than in girls.

Life in the Womb and Schizophrenia

It was the tragic Dutch Hunger Winter that taught us the most about how life in the womb can increase the risk of developing schizophrenia. A large, multifaceted research study helped us understand how conditions in the womb might affect the risk for schizophrenia.

A large amount of evidence gives us good knowledge that poor prenatal nutrition is a very pivotal factor in causing birth defects of the spinal column and brain, spina bifida being perhaps the most well known example of such defects. (As you'll learn later in this book, a deficiency of folic acid, a B vitamin, is thought to cause a significant percentage of spinal column defects.) Thus, it was logical to look into the possibility that poor prenatal nutrition might cause abnormalities in brain structure and function that can lead to the constellation of symptoms known as schizophrenia. The behavior of a person diagnosed with schizophrenia is characterized by disordered thinking that includes hallucinations (for example, a person might see spiders crawling on her skin when really there are none present), delusions (believing that something is true that is not; someone might believe that he is Napoleon, for example), and other problems with reality-based thinking.

It was a research team led by Dr. Ezra Susser that delved deeply into the effects of poor nutrition on schizophrenic disorders. As you learned earlier, it was Ezra Susser's parents who first made the connection between poor nutrition in the womb and health in adulthood.

About 40,000 babies exposed to famine at some point in gestation were born during or after the Hunger Winter. As you read earlier, the clear demarcation of the famine in time and place provided good information regarding who was suffering from inadequate in utero nutrition and during which stages of their prenatal development the undernourishment occurred. In other words, any individual could be identified as being malnourished during early, middle, or late gestation—or more than one of these periods. The researchers also had knowledge of those people who had schizophrenic conditions many decades later and they compared the incidence of schizophrenia among the individuals who were malnourished in utero with the incidence among people who were born in the same cities where the famine occurred but who either were born in the time period just before or were conceived after it ended.

The researchers found an increased incidence of schizophrenia among the people conceived at the height of the famine and subsequent birth defects of the nervous system. The risk of schizophrenia clearly peaked in the people who experienced famine while in their mother's womb. Both men and women who experienced famine in utero during the Dutch Hunger Winter were about twice as likely to have schizophrenia as their comrades who did not develop in the womb under famine conditions. Further analysis, this time separating those people who were conceived at the peak of the famine, found an even greater increase in schizophrenia; their risk was increased nearly threefold.

In another aspect of their research, investigators studied whether famine in utero also increased the risk of schizoid personality disorder, which includes a broader spectrum of symptoms associated with schizophrenia. They found that the risk for the famine-exposed men (they studied only men) was slightly more than doubled by the time they reached 18 years of age.

Research Recap

- **Fetal origins of chronic disease describes the long-lasting effects of either positive or negative conditions at a sensitive or critical period of development of a baby's organs, tissues, and other body systems while a baby is in the womb. Epidemiologists are working to find relations between life in the womb and future risk of disease.**
- **Undernourishment early in pregnancy, when the baby's body organs are forming, may increase risk of central nervous system birth defects, such as spina bifida, and double the likelihood of developing schizophrenia.**

(continued)

Research Recap (continued)

- Babies born full term but underweight have an increased risk of developing cardiovascular disease (both coronary artery disease and stroke) than do those with a higher birth weight.
- Babies who are undernourished during their first trimester are far more likely to become overweight as adults than are those who are properly nourished; on the other hand, babies who are overfed in the womb towards the end of gestation and born too heavy also have a significantly increased risk of adult weight problems.
- Low birth weight may increase the chances of abdominal obesity in adulthood, which in turn is associated with greater risk of diseases such as heart disease, diabetes, and hypertension.
- There is an association between birth weight and breast cancer risk in women: the higher the birth weight, the higher the frequency of breast cancer.
- Preliminary data suggest that the smaller the abdomen at birth, the higher the cholesterol levels in adult life.
- Undernourishment in late pregnancy may increase the risk of asthma, as does maternal smoking.
- Men whose birth weight was 8.7 pounds or greater at birth were five times more likely to develop prostate cancer compared with men who weighed less than 8.7 pounds.
- Men who, when born, weighed between 5.5 and 8.8 pounds, have a decreased risk of developing testicular cancer as adults compared with those whose birth weight was below 5.5 pounds or above 8.8 pounds.
- Children whose birth weight was more than 9.9 pounds had a 70% increased risk of developing acute lymphatic leukemia compared to those who weighed less than 9.9 pounds; high birth weight may also increase the risk of other types of leukemia.
- Brain cancer risk is about 2.5 times as great in children under the age of 14 who were born weighing more than 8 pounds at birth compared with those who weighed less than 8 pounds.

PRENATAL LIFE AND OTHER CONDITIONS

There is also mounting evidence that the prenatal environment influences a person's risk of several other conditions and affects other body systems, including cholesterol levels. For example, there is preliminary evidence that the smaller the abdomen at birth, the higher the cholesterol level in adult life.

BEYOND BIRTH WEIGHT

Indeed, birth weight is an important predictor of your child's future health. But as birth weight is just a marker in the link between conditions in the womb and the long term health of your child, we scientists are looking to find other traces that help us to understand the relation between mom's diet and baby's long-term health more directly.

Our new research takes us beyond the birth weight observations. We know that it's not just the number of calories and the amount of weight a woman gains, but the quality of her diet or the types of foods she eats is emerging as ever more important.

These "precious" and exciting links between an expectant mom's diet and her child's risk of disease later in life can sometimes even be completely independent of her baby's size at birth. These are the links, based on scientific evidence that I want to share here.

The first one returns to the observations made during the Dutch Famine winter of 1944–1945, which was mentioned earlier. The children born to women who were malnourished early in the pregnancy suffered many consequences as adults. Some of them seem to work via the birth-weight route, others seem to operate directly, independent of the children's birthweight.

For one, we now know that the children of women pregnant during this grim period often have, in their adult life, what is technically called a lower glucose tolerance. This means that their bodies do not respond normally to sugar in the bloodstream. As a result, they are at much higher risk for developing type 2 diabetes mellitus in middle age and beyond, and possibly even sooner if they become overweight and/or sedentary.

Another ill effect of children deprived nutritionally during the first trimester of pregnancy that shows up in adult life is an abnormality in blood fats. The most common blood fat is cholesterol: research has now shown us that when cholesterol levels were measured around age 50, they had too-high levels of bad cholesterol (officially known as low density lipoprotein or LDL-cholesterol) and too-low levels of good cholesterol (high density lipoprotein, HDL-cholesterol) as compared to other men and women of the same age whose mothers were well nourished during their pregnancy. These effects were found to be independent of birth weight. (Incidentally, these abnormal levels of blood fats were also independent of adult obesity, which is a known risk factor for this problem.)

David Barker's group in England made other observations between a mother-to-be's eating habits and her child's adult health. Studying a Scottish population, Barker's group found that when mom ate an unbalanced diet during pregnancy, her child was more likely to have high blood pressure as an adult. Specifically, Barker found that if mom consumed a diet very high in carbohydrate and too low in protein, as well as vice versa: a diet that is too low in carbohydrate and too high in protein, during late pregnancy, the offspring were more likely to have elevated blood pressure at age 40. Again, this observation was independent of calorie intake during pregnancy.

Greek researchers have found some evidence that quality of the mom's diet during pregnancy may impact the risk of cerebral palsy in the child. Mothers in the Greater Athens area who gave birth to children with cerebral palsy were asked about what they ate during pregnancy. Compared with mothers of healthy children, the mothers of children with cerebral palsy had consumed considerably more meat and eggs and less fish during their pregnancy.

The last thing I would like to discuss relates to my area of interest: breast cancer. While data on maternal diet and the risk of breast cancer in the daughter are not yet available for humans, interesting observations have been made in study animals. For example, in rodent studies, the female offspring born to mothers fed a very high fat diet (43% of calories) during the entire pregnancy had a much higher chance of developing breast cancer when they were exposed to known cancer-causing substances. In these studies, the rodents were fed a specific type of oil, corn oil. The type of oil may be significant. Corn oil consists mainly of linoleic acid, a type of oil that increases levels of the hormone estradiol. We suspect that the consumption of the oil was sufficient to raise hormones and expose the fetuses to elevated estradiol levels. In these studies, it was also noted that the female offspring had earlier onset puberty (yes, rodents have a defined puberty, too!). In addition, the cells of their breasts were slightly abnormal, which made them more susceptible to becoming cancerous.

What I would like you to take away from all of this is that while we want you to eat an appropriate number of calories during your pregnancy, we also want to make sure you eat a healthy and well-balanced diet. That's why you'll see very specific foods and recipes in our meal plans. We've done our best to translate the science into food—and delicious at that—that you can put on your plate each and every day with a tremendous peace of mind that you are doing the best you can to nourish your baby in the womb—and for his or her good health throughout life. While olive oil is the primary source of fat in Southern European populations who have the world's highest longevity, some other fats—in small amounts—may also be of value. These can be found in soybeans, walnuts, flaxseed and flaxseed oil, canola oil and fish, especially salmon, mackerel, tuna, and trout.

PUTTING ALL OF THIS RESEARCH INTO PERSPECTIVE

After reading this evidence, I want to reemphasize one very important point: *Fetal origins of chronic disease is only one of several factors that may determine your child-to-be's adult health risks.* Although the conditions in the womb are an important factor, genetics and lifestyle also have a tremendous impact on how fetal influences play out. I believe in the life course approach, which stresses the full range of physical, emotional, and environmental issues that affect a person's life, from the time in the womb through the teen and adult years. So if you have already had one (or more) children or if you are already into your pregnancy, don't worry:

Fetal Origins in Perspective

I want to emphasize something I mentioned in the Introduction. As critical as it may be, the fetal origin of disease theory does not operate in a vacuum. Instead, it is one factor in a person's whole life course. *Life course* is a term used by researchers of the fetal origins hypothesis to describe the full range of physical, behavioral, and environmental hazards throughout the course of a person's life that impacts his or her health status and disease risk. The life course actually begins at the moment of conception, when a person's genetic makeup is determined. Then, life in the womb adds its signature.

(continued)

Fetal Origins in Perspective (continued)

After birth, a person's care during infancy and on into childhood leaves yet another imprint on what will eventually emerge as adulthood health status. Did you know, for example, that even young children could begin to develop the "sludge" in their arteries that we know as atherosclerosis? Lifestyle habits from childhood on into adulthood then greatly impact how both genetics and fetal conditioning play out. Let's take a look at Frank, a man quite unlike Margaret, who was mentioned earlier. Certain events in Frank's life eventually led to his suffering a heart attack at the age of 57:

- Being overweight since he was a teenager
- Eating a diet high in saturated and *trans*-fatty acids, refined sugars, and carbohydrates from the time he was a child
- Smoking from the time he was 19 years old
- Having a father with early-onset heart disease (he suffered a heart attack at age 43) and a paternal grandfather who died of a stroke at age 56
- Living a sedentary life—not exercising much beyond walking from the car to his office

Even though he had a strong family history of heart disease, Frank might never have developed it himself (nor had a heart attack) if he had had different *life course events*. If he had lived an active life, eaten a healthier diet, and not smoked, he might have been able to counter his family history—alias his genes.

I hope this example helps you appreciate even more that a person's whole life is important in determining disease risk, not just single factors such as the fetal environment or family history. Indeed, although Margaret couldn't seem to overcome her early life course events, Frank might have been able to. Although this seems contradictory, it actually illustrates well that every aspect of people's lives, from their genetics and their days in the womb to childhood, teen, and adult life issues, can indeed determine their health in their later years.

There are many things you can do today and tomorrow to promote the good health of your children.

Please remember, too, that although what you do during your pregnancy is very important, you shouldn't try to influence birth weight to *the extreme*. Never overindulge or starve yourself in an attempt to control your baby's birth weight. As you have learned while reading through this chapter, birth weight seems to be an important marker of prenatal events. But as we also know now, different birth weight levels affect the risk of chronic disease in different ways. For instance, birth weight *is* related to both cardiovascular disease and breast cancer but in *opposite* ways: Whereas babies born very heavy may have a lower risk of heart disease and stroke, they also may have a higher chance of experiencing cancer in later life.

This is why my best advice to you is to achieve the middle road, gain the recommended amount of weight (25 to 35 pounds) during your pregnancy, follow the guidelines in this book, and always concentrate on maintaining good eating habits as best you can.

Now, please read on for more details on how you can help your baby and child-to-be from this moment forward. You'll begin to see that moms make a huge difference—throughout their offsprings' life!

CHAPTER TWO

From Heart Disease to Diabetes

The Impact of Diet and Other Factors
on Specific Diseases

Now that you have an idea that life in the womb can affect your baby-to-be in his or her adult life, I would like to explain how this happens.

The mechanisms by which conditions in the womb impact the adult health of the child you are about to have are subtle. Indeed, they are far subtler than the ones we traditionally associate with affecting an unborn baby. For example, you've probably heard a lot of the immediate effects of tobacco, alcohol, and certain drugs on a developing baby. By immediate, I mean the factors we notice at birth. A baby exposed to cigarette smoke in utero, for example, may be born much smaller than expected and is also at higher risk of being born with a cleft lip or palate. Babies exposed to alcohol during their developing days in the womb can be born with a con-stellation of very characteristic physical and intellectual disabilities called fetal alcohol syndrome. Exposure to certain drugs such as cocaine and specific prescription or over-the-counter medications can cause profound birth defects or addiction at birth.

But the science of fetal origins deals with far less blatant effects. Yes, as you read in Chapter One, there may be immediate indications, such as low birth weight, telling us that growth conditions in the womb were not optimal. But experts on fetal origins have learned that these immediate factors may just be a marker for other, more consequential changes that happen in utero. When conditions aren't optimal for growth—such as

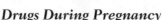

Drugs During Pregnancy

The list of both prescription and over-the-counter drugs grows nearly daily. Although some of these are safe for pregnant women, others are not. Because we could never provide you with a constantly up-to-date list of all potentially dangerous medications, we think it is better to advise you to ask your obstetrician or midwife about medications. Before you take anything—from vitamin supplements and herbs to prescription medications and laxatives—check first with your health-care provider.

when the calorie or nutrient supply isn't adequate—this often means that there are alterations in womb chemistry. Fetal origins research is based on the theory that these subtle changes in womb chemistry might have a profound and long-lasting effect on the baby's own chemistry, and thus on his or her developing cells and tissues.

In this chapter, I'll first describe the ways a mother's nutrition impacts her baby during his or her time in the womb and at birth. Then I'll walk you through the conditions I discussed in Chapter One and explain the mechanisms of the interactions between mom and her unborn baby that seem to increase the risk of these illnesses in adulthood. I'll also tell you how optimal nutrition during pregnancy can help reduce the chance of their occurrence in your unborn child, many decades into his or her future.

How a Healthy Diet Benefits You and Baby

Who ever thought eating would carry such big responsibilities? Although eating in a healthful manner at every stage of life is important, it is even more consequential during your days in waiting.

The child inside of you (or the one soon to be there) is totally dependent on you. He or she gets all nutrients and calories from your body. You probably already know by now that your baby grows inside of a wonderfully safe cocoon called the placenta. Many people also call it the womb. The placenta develops inside your uterus after conception; after baby's birth, you also deliver the placenta.

The placenta is a blood- and nutrient-rich sac that cushions your baby from the bounces and bumps he or she takes every day as you move about, jog, or perhaps get elbowed by a little one or by a fellow shopper in a busy store. (The placenta is filled with amniotic fluid, which provides another wonderful cushioning effect for baby.)

For the placenta to grow and nourish baby, mom must "feed" the placenta. The placenta must grow in size as the baby grows. During gestation, if nutrition is suboptimal, the baby has an incredible ability to prioritize where the limited amounts of nutrients and/or calories go. If you think about it, this is actually a wonderful survival mechanism: Without a properly developed brain, a child might not be able to function physically, emotionally, or mentally in the world. This is why baby's developing brain is always served first. In times of suboptimal nutrition, baby's brain will be supplied at the expense of other organs. As you read the details of how nutrition impacts life in the womb and then baby's future risk of disease, you will understand in greater detail the impact of this phenomenon.

Although reproduction experts have always known that the placenta needs good nutrition to grow properly and therefore allow baby to develop optimally, the effects were never quantified until recently. In 1996, Dr. Barker and his colleagues at the Medical Research Council Environmental Epidemiology Unit at the University of Southampton in England set out to quantify this association. In their research, they kept track of three sets of data. One was the mother's diet during pregnancy. A second was placental weight at birth. The third was birth weight according to the sex of the baby (birth weight varies by sex) and length of gestation (a shorter gestation, or being born before 40 weeks' gestation, results in a smaller baby and a smaller placenta).

Dr. Barker's team found that not just adequate calories but also optimal nutrition affected the weight of the placenta. Mothers with high carbohydrate and low protein intake in early pregnancy delivered both babies and placentas that were of lower-than-average weight. Moms who had low intakes of protein in late pregnancy also gave birth to lighter-than-average babies and placentas. In both cases, the associations were independent of the mother's height and prepregnancy BMI.

The bottom line is that eating well—obtaining the optimal amount of all nutrients and of total calories—is essential to help the placenta and the baby grow optimally.

Now let's see how nutrition is thought to impact each of the diseases I discussed in Chapter One.

Birth Weight and Prematurity: What's the Difference?

As you read through the information in this chapter, you'll learn a lot about both low and high birth weight as they relate to certain conditions. I'd like you to remember one critical detail about low and high birth weight that I broached in Chapter One: The reason for low birth weight is very important in sorting out the impact it can make on the baby at birth, and the effect it can have on health as that child grows into an adult.

There are two different types of low birth weight. One involves babies who are born with a low birth weight simply because they are born too early, or prematurely. If they had been born at the appropriate time—if they were left to finish growing in mom's womb to full term—many of these babies would have been born at an optimal birth weight. Then there is the group of babies born at term but smaller than the expected norm. In this group of newborns, there was something about life in the womb that wasn't quite right. For some reason, they didn't receive optimal nutrition and so couldn't grow to the healthiest weight range. In most cases, this latter group is the one we are talking about.

The prematurely born babies, however, often compensate for their smallness at birth by trying to catch up to their peers during the first few years of life. To do so, they produce high amounts of growth hormones that, in turn, may lead to high blood pressure and might also promote the growth of cancer cells.

CARDIOVASCULAR DISEASE

As you already read, low birth weight is thought to increase the risk of atherosclerosis (also called cardiovascular disease or heart disease) in adult life. More specifically, though, low birth weight increases the chances that a person will develop the risk factors that lead to atherosclerosis. Two of the most important risk factors are hypertension, or high blood pressure, and high blood cholesterol levels. These are the factors we will discuss as we explain how life in the womb can impact a baby's adult risk of heart disease.

The Origins of Hypertension

There are several theories why low birth weight may increase the risk of adult hypertension. The first theory is simply about growth—when a baby doesn't grow optimally in utero, it is possible that certain tissues don't grow properly, either. As we mentioned above, when there is limited nutrition, it goes preferentially to the baby's developing brain. In turn, other tissues may not grow optimally. Although many tissues might be adversely affected, those that may affect hypertension are the kidneys and the blood vessels.

A person's kidneys have a tremendous impact on blood pressure. This is because the body depends on the kidneys to filter out just the right amount of fluid from the body. If too much fluid stays in the body, a condition called fluid retention, it raises blood pressure. Conversely, if the kidneys filter out too much fluid, blood pressure drops too much, which can cause a person to become dizzy or to faint.

Kidneys are formed of small components called nephrons. A person with normal kidneys has somewhere between 300,000 and 1 million nephrons. People who do not have normal numbers of nephrons have abnormally high levels of pressure in the capillaries, or small blood vessels, that form the nephrons. In turn, the high pressure damages and then hardens the walls of the capillaries. The result: people with hardening of the capillary walls in the nephrons cannot filter out fluid normally. Thus, they have a much more difficult time controlling blood pressure.

Nephrons are formed during fetal life. Both human and animal studies have taught us that babies who do not grow optimally during fetal life also have abnormally low numbers of nephrons. Ultrasound studies of developing babies have provided more evidence that kidney growth is compromised in babies who do not develop normally. Today most women have a fetal ultrasound as part of their routine prenatal care; sometimes, however, obstetricians order them when they suspect mom's abdomen is not growing at the appropriate rate (at each prenatal visit, the doctor or midwife measures the abdomen—this is officially called the fundal height) or when she isn't gaining enough weight. (See "Fetal Ultrasound," page 43). Combined data from large numbers of ultrasound studies on babies who are not growing properly have shown that such babies have decreased kidney growth during the critical period of 26 to 34 weeks (about 6.5 to 8 months) of gestation when nephron numbers generally increase the most.

Fetal Ultrasound

Fetal ultrasound gives obstetricians the ability to look inside the womb. Ultrasound, performed by a radiologist, an ultrasound technician, or an obstetrician, is a technique that uses sound waves to create an image. A picture of the baby growing inside the womb is generated as the sound waves bounce off the different tissues in the mother's abdomen, including the baby. Early in pregnancy, you may be instructed to drink lots of water and to arrive at your ultrasound appointment with a full bladder. The reason? A full bladder may be needed to push the bowel out of the way in the abdomen, which helps in providing an unobstructed view of the developing baby. Ultrasound technology does not use any radiation, so there is no need to worry about the safety. In addition to checking on the development of the baby, obstetricians use ultrasound to determine your due date, especially if you are not sure about the date of your last period and when you became pregnant.

Another theory about how suboptimal nutrition in fetal life can lead to adult hypertension is that it may limit the normal development of the baby's blood vessel system. This may be traceable to the development of one of the most important arteries in the body, the aorta. The aorta is the large blood vessel attached to the top of the heart. It is through the aorta that blood leaves the heart after it is oxygenated; the aorta branches out to all the vessels that supply blood to the rest of the body. This is how oxygen is delivered to all the cells of the body.

The aorta has to be very elastic to control how much blood flows to the rest of the body. When the aorta is not elastic, the chance of high blood pressure is increased. Elasticity is determined in large part by a protein called elastin. This protein is deposited into arteries in utero and during infancy. Studies have shown, however, that babies with a low birth weight deposit far less elastin into their arteries during their time in the womb than do their higher-weight counterparts. Unlike many other proteins, elastin turns over, or is replaced, very slowly: At 40 years of age, just about half of this protein will have been replaced from the original proteins present at birth. So, when decreased amounts of elastin are laid down during fetal life, the arteries are less elastic throughout life. The situation is compounded as a person ages. As we age, all body proteins, including elastin, stiffen. So the less elastin there is to begin with, the earlier blood vessels will stiffen—and the earlier a person will develop hypertension.

The endocrine, or hormone, system of the body also affects blood pressure in a number of ways, and conditions in the womb are thought to impact several hormone systems. The endocrine system produces many hormones, including cortisol. When present in the body at excessive levels, cortisol can raise blood pressure. The impact of excessive cortisol levels may begin in the womb, say experts in the field of the fetal origins of disease. When fetal conditions are optimal, an enzyme (a protein that acts like a chemical knife to break apart body chemicals) deactivates cortisol so that it does not build up in the body. However, when mom does not get optimal nutrition—most especially, when she doesn't get enough protein—her placenta cannot make enough properly functioning anticortisol enzymes. As a result, higher-than-normal levels of cortisol reach the fetal brain. Scientists who study fetal origins of disease believe that a fetus exposed to excessive levels of cortisol has an increased sensitivity to this hormone. This means that the baby's body becomes conditioned to overreact to cortisol. A fetus exposed to high cortisol levels may be more susceptible to it and therefore to hypertension throughout life.

The kidneys produce a hormone called renin, which also contributes to blood pressure control. Research suggests that suboptimal growth in the womb causes the fetal kidneys to produce extra renin. Scientists think that this higher level of renin exerts a very early and long-lasting influence, increasing the likelihood of high blood pressure as an adult.

A growth hormone called insulin-like growth factor–1 (IGF-1) also elevates blood pressure when it is present in the body at higher-than-normal levels. Children born with a low birth weight tend to have abnormally high levels of IGF-1. The highest levels are found in children who had very low birth weights but grew very fast during the first 1 or 2 years of life. When children are very small at birth and then grow rapidly during their first 2 years of life, we say that they undergo *catch-up growth*. This ability to catch up, or to compensate for slower growth in the womb, may be programmed in utero.

Undernourished fetuses may try to compensate by making more IGF-1 than do babies who are better nourished. Having this enhanced production of IGF-1 apparently improves a child's ability for catch-up growth when nutrition is better. There is a downside, however, to this enhanced

IGF-1 production. In the case of IGF-1, experts on blood pressure know that people who produce more IGF have a lifelong tendency toward higher blood pressure. Interestingly, we are also speculating that high IGF-1 levels may also be associated with future breast cancer risk.

The Origins of Cholesterol Levels

A baby in the womb has an amazing ability to survive, even when he or she cannot get enough nutrition. When food is scarce, the baby's growing body prioritizes which of its developing tissues and organs will get what's provided. In other words, the fetus shifts into emergency mode. Because the brain is the most vital organ, blood and the nutrients it supplies are preferentially shuttled there, as we explained previously.

When food is scarce, organs in the abdomen get the leftovers. These organs can include the liver. Research has shown that babies born smaller than average are more likely to have livers that are also smaller than normal.

Among other jobs, the liver plays a very important role in regulating blood cholesterol levels. Cells in the liver have something akin to large grappling hooks that snare cholesterol from the blood and send it out of the body through the digestive tract. Smaller livers have fewer liver cells. In turn, this means that people with smaller livers have fewer grappling hooks—and a reduced ability to clear cholesterol from the blood. This may be an important factor in why some people who eat wisely—a low-fat, low-cholesterol diet—still have trouble with their blood cholesterol levels, whereas other people can eat French fries and bacon with reckless abandon and still maintain a low blood cholesterol level. Of course, genetics, or your mother's and father's tendencies to have high cholesterol levels, plays an important role as well.

ADULT WEIGHT

The effects of fetal life on adult weight illustrate well the importance of just the right conditions in the womb. Depending on the timing, a baby who develops in a womb that doesn't supply enough nutrition is more likely to become obese as an adult. But we know that babies who develop in conditions of excess—when mom takes in too many calories—also have a much greater chance of battling weight problems as an adult.

Researchers think that when calories are scarce during the first trimester, a baby learns to be very thrifty—developing a thrifty phenotype. This means that the baby learns to hang on to every calorie it encounters, never knowing if more will come along. These metabolically efficient babies also learn to use fewer calories to grow and develop and also to store any excess calories with the utmost efficiency. Unfortunately, this thrifty metabolism seems to stick for life, even when calories aren't so scarce.

There is another theory why babies who have grown under famine conditions in the womb are predisposed to adult weight problems. It is possible that babies undernourished during their first trimester in the womb have a permanent change in the appetite control center of their brains. Specifically, the appetite control center may be set into overdrive permanently. Having once known famine, the appetite control panel may be programmed with the philosophy that "you never know when food is going to be available, so eat whatever is around, when it is around." Like a thrifty metabolism, this appetite change may operate for life, even when it is not necessary.

Worse than having a thrifty metabolism or an appetite in constant over-drive, is being saddled with both because of developing in a womb that did not have enough calories, protein, and/or nutrients.

On the other side of the coin, too many calories during the last months of life in the womb are not favorable, either. Babies growing inside of a mom who consumes too many calories (and not necessarily many too many calories) may make more than the normal number of fat cells. Babies born with extra fat cells—alias heavier babies—are more likely to fill those fat cells and become overweight as adults.

DIABETES MELLITUS

As I discussed in Chapter One, being born very small increases a child's likelihood of developing diabetes mellitus in later life. To understand how conditions in the womb can increase the risk for this type of diabetes, let me first explain a little bit about this condition.

About Blood Sugars

Simply put, diabetes is a blood sugar problem: People with diabetes cannot control their blood sugars as nature intended, and so may have elevated levels of "sugar" in their bloodstream. Glucose comes from food, which the body breaks down and digests to its simplest form, glucose. The glucose is then absorbed into the bloodstream. Every one of us must always have some glucose in our bloodstream. It's the fuel that's used by every cell in the body and the brain. When cells use up their available stores of glucose, they quickly get replenished with the glucose that's floating nearby in the blood.

It's normal for glucose levels to periodically spike after meals. These temporary elevations of glucose are normal and aren't likely to cause problems for most people. However, a different picture emerges when glucose levels are persistently high. When this happens, the glucose literally becomes toxic. This may create serious complications if it isn't quickly restored to normal levels.

The damage begins in the blood vessels. Over time, high levels of glucose may damage tissues in the capillaries, the tiny vessels that carry blood and oxygen to the body's cells. The capillaries in the eyes are especially susceptible; people with diabetes have a high risk of developing an eye disease called retinopathy, which occurs when capillaries in the eyes leak or rupture. Also at risk are blood vessels in the kidneys or feet.

More serious still, people with diabetes have a high risk of developing heart disease, in part because glucose-ravaged blood vessels may interfere with circulation and raise blood pressure to dangerous levels.

Where Does Blood Glucose Come From?

Glucose is just one of a number of different types of sugars, also known as carbohydrates. Some carbohydrates, including glucose, are known as simple sugars or simple carbohydrates because they are made of only one or two sugar units. These simple sugars are found in sweet foods such as soda and table sugar. Others are termed complex carbohydrates because they are made of many sugar units linked together, sometimes hundreds of them. These nonsweet forms of carbohydrate are often called starches and are familiar to us in the form of foods such as whole-grain bread and brown rice.

Although not much of the carbohydrate we eat is in the form of simple glucose units, our bodies will eventually convert all of it to glucose, as this is the form the body prefers for fuel. When it

(continued)

Where Does Blood Glucose Come From? (continued)

comes to digestion, however, simple and complex carbohydrates are digested differently. The long chains of sugar units found in complex carbohydrates or starch are composed of glucose units linked together. When they enter the digestive system, the body's digestive juices split off the glucose units one by one, so the body absorbs them slowly. Simple sugar units found in sweet foods such as candy can be absorbed quickly, on the other hand, because they are already in small "packages," having only one or two sugar units. In other words, the simple sugars will enter the bloodstream much more quickly than will the glucose from complex carbohydrates and can cause a steeper increase in blood glucose in people with diabetes. You can understand, then, why diabetes experts recommend consuming the majority of carbohydrate or sugar calories in the complex form. (The other reasons have to do with the fact that complex carbohydrates also contain infinitely more vitamins, minerals, and fibers.)

Interestingly, breaking down protein and even fat from foods we eat yields some glucose. Although 100% of all carbohydrates eventually yields glucose, just 58% of protein is converted into glucose and a mere 10% of fat becomes glucose. In addition, this "disassembly" process of protein and fat foods into their building blocks (which includes some glucose) takes much longer than breaking down carbohydrate. This is why diabetes doctors are so keen on people with diabetes dividing their calories appropriately among carbohydrates, proteins, and fats.

Controlling Blood Sugars

The body was created with an incredible ability to regulate blood glucose. The main control mechanism? Insulin. The pancreas produces insulin, which is a hormone. Insulin is like a key, unlocking the door of the body's cells to let the glucose in. Only when glucose leaves the bloodstream and enters the cells can the body make use of it: Once inside the cells, glucose is either burned for energy or stored for later use.

When the body's very sensitive information system registers an increase in blood sugar levels, it sends a message to the pancreas to pump out more insulin, which lets glucose inside cells. People with diabetes, however, have problems responding to this message. In some cases, their body may not be able to produce the extra insulin. In others, the body makes the needed insulin, but the body's cells do not respond to it and don't let the extra glucose in. In medicine, we say that the body is insensitive (or resistant) to insulin.

A host of very complicated factors predict whether a diabetic person's body is appropriately sensitive to insulin, including whether they are overweight and if they have a genetic predisposition to diabetes. The amount of muscle is another very important predictive factor. Muscle mass helps insulin work more effectively—it increases the body's sensitivity to insulin, meaning that the body can more quickly move sugar from the blood into the cells, thereby avoiding elevated blood sugar readings.

How Fetal Life May Affect Diabetes Risk

Experts on fetal origins of disease believe there are at least a couple of reasons why certain suboptimal nutritional conditions in the womb can increase the rise of type 2 diabetes. Suboptimal nutrition can mean too few calories or less than optimal diet composition, such as not enough protein or not enough nutrients.

Studies have shown that people born at smaller-than-average birth weights have reduced muscle mass. This tends to be the result of decreased nutrition in midgestation (the middle months of pregnancy). These middle months of pregnancy are the prime time for the baby to develop muscle bulk.

Another reason why too few calories during gestation may increase the risk for diabetes has to do with the fetus's survival response. When calories are scarce, the developing baby learns to decrease its dependence on glucose for the energy it needs to grow. Instead, the baby turns to other fuel sources, including amino acids, the building blocks of protein that are always floating around in the bloodstream. When conditions are very sparse, the baby may even break down the muscle tissue it has already built up to use for energy. As you've just read, less muscle mass may, in itself, lead to an increased risk of diabetes in later life.

The problem with turning to these other energy sources is that the cells may get rusty at shuttling glucose into the cells. We think that babies growing in conditions of too few calories might permanently lose some of their ability to transfer glucose from the bloodstream into cells, leading to higher levels of glucose circulating in the blood. If mom has diabetes during pregnancy that is not controlled, her baby may also have a greater-than-normal risk of developing diabetes as a child or an adult. Although some women have diabetes before they become pregnant, others develop gestational diabetes, or pregnancy-induced diabetes, during pregnancy. Gestational diabetes can develop in any woman, but it is more likely to develop in women who are heavier than average before pregnancy. Because avoiding high blood sugars during pregnancy is so important, we have devoted a whole chapter, Chapter Nine, to this issue.

Reducing Your Future Child's Adult Risk of Diabetes

The actions you can take to reduce your child's adult risk of developing diabetes begin with starting your pregnancy at an optimal weight. If you are heavier than the average weight for your height (or if you have a body mass index [BMI] greater than 29—see pages 65–66) and you are not yet pregnant, try to drop some weight before you conceive. We have devoted a whole chapter to how to eat before you become pregnant, Chapter Five. Once you do become pregnant, concentrate on gaining just the right amount of weight, which means feeding the baby inside of you with just the right number of calories each and every day.

BREAST CANCER

In Chapter One, I told you the exciting story of my discovery of the relation between lower birth weight and a reduced risk of breast cancer. Now, how do we explain these startling findings on a cellular level? What mechanisms may be behind this association? Birth weight itself is likely only a reflection of the conditions and processes in the womb that affect breast cancer risk, rather than the actual cause of the disease.

Scientists, including me, believe that the mother's hormonal levels are probably a very important factor. As you would realize, during pregnancy your hormones change dramatically. In particular, growth hormones, a group that includes the important hormones estrogen and IGF-1, increase dramatically. This is because there is a little human being growing inside you. The tiny breast cells of a baby girl in the womb are exposed to all these growth hormones, more that they will ever be exposed to again during life after birth. Unfortunately, at this time the breast cells are very vulnerable to external influences because they are what scientists call undifferentiated. Not until decades later when that girl is grown and pregnant will the breast cells undergo changes to take up their primary function: lactation. You can read more about breast cell differentiation below. Just keep in mind that this means that the cells are very susceptible to the influence of hormones when they are undifferentiated.

Breast Cell Differentiation

Think of undifferentiated cells as a group of trainees in a car factory on their first day of work. None of them knows on that first day which specific task they will be trained to do. But eventually, they all will be assigned a certain task and they will be trained to perform that task. Only because they all acquire the skills and work together can the final product, the car, be built.

Breast cells are similarly "trained." In the beginning, they are a mass of undifferentiated, unspecific cells that could develop into any kind of breast cell. They have not learned yet what their precise function will be later in life—just that they will be "grownup" breast cells one day. During puberty, they grow and divide further. But it is only once a woman gets pregnant that her breast cells find their true calling: to take up some of the specific functions to aid the lactation process, from forming the lining of the ducts that will carry the breast milk to grouping around the ends of the ducts where the milk is produced, and so on. The cells have then differentiated into various types of breast cells that can take on the many processes involved in the production of breast milk.

The way estrogen and other growth hormones work is by inducing cells to divide more frequently. Each time a cell divides, there is a very small chance that an error can occur in the transcription of the genetic code, or DNA (deoxyribonucleic acid). These errors, in turn, lead to a very small chance that cancer could occur in later life. Thus, the higher the levels of growth hormones, the more frequently the breast cells divide, and the more the risk of cancer, however small, increases. Of course, although the breast tissue is particularly susceptible to these hormones, increased levels of growth factors will lead to a bigger baby overall, thus the relations between higher birth weights and breast cancer risk.

Recently, Dr. Anders Ekbom made a very interesting observation: Baby girls born very prematurely were at an increased risk of breast cancer—in particular those with very low birth weight. While this seems a paradox at first, there may be a very plausible explanation for this phenomenon. During the first couple of years of their postnatal life, these preemies are trying to catch up to their peers who were born at term. This means they grow at an accelerated pace and they get help from the most potent growth factor, IGF-1. As we discussed, rapid growth increases the chance of genetic errors when cells divide, resulting in a greater risk of developing breast cancer.

This leads us to the question of how our levels of estrogen and other growth factors are determined. Part of the answer is: We don't exactly know. There is a great variation in natural levels of these hormones, and two women of the same height and weight may have quite different levels, probably due partly to genetics. Controlling weight and total calorie intake are other factors that influence levels of growth hormones. This is one of the reasons we recommend controlling the amount of weight you gain during pregnancy. Gaining excessive weight can make your baby grow more quickly and become larger than average. Chapter Three will outline the recommended rates of weight gain for each trimester. A healthy, well-balanced diet of an appropriate number of calories, such as the Optimal Pregnancy Diet in this book, will translate into optimal growth of your baby and thus provide her (or him) with the best possible starting point for a long and healthy life.

Expectant moms often wonder if there is any way to prevent their babies from experiencing cancer. As we have stressed throughout this book so far, eating a certain nutrient or a specific number of calories doesn't directly decrease or increase your child's future risk of disease. Rather, optimizing your nutrition is the best way to improve your child's growth, which is what probably helps reduce the disease risk. We do this with the Optimal Pregnancy Diet. With respect to breast cancer, eating the right amount of calories with an abundance of good nutrients can help set a more optimal hormonal environment for your baby and thus may help her lower her chances of developing breast cancer as an adult woman.

PROSTATE AND TESTICULAR CANCER

In Chapter One, you learned that baby boys born heavier than average may have an increased risk of developing both prostate and testicular cancer when they become adults. You also learned that male babies born heavier or lighter than average may have an increased risk of testicular cancer. As it turns out, there are two types of testicular cancer, and one type, testicular seminomas, is more common among men with high birth weight, whereas testicular nonseminomas were found more often among men born light.

The underlying mechanism for both prostate cancer and testicular seminomas could be similar to that proposed for breast cancer. Growth hormones operate in utero to help the baby grow. The most powerful growth hormone operating during prenatal life is IGF-1. High IGF-1 levels in the blood of the baby may make it grow faster and bigger, in turn increasing the possibilities for genetic mutations as described for breast cancer above.

Unfortunately, our knowledge about what influences a baby's level of growth hormones is limited. The best you can do is control your body weight and excessive calorie intake.

PRENATAL LIFE AND CHILDHOOD CANCERS

You learned in Chapter One that being born heavier than normal increases the risk of several types of leukemia common to children, including acute lymphatic leukemia, acute lymphoblastic leukemia (ALL), and acute myeloid leukemia (AML). Researchers have also found that babies born to mothers who had high blood pressure, or maternal hypertension, have an increased risk of developing acute lymphatic leukemia. Brain cancer, the second most common childhood cancer, also occurs at a higher rate in children who were born with a higher-than-average birth weight.

What is it about conditions of excess in the womb that might increase childhood cancer risk, ask researchers. As with the other types of cancer discussed in this chapter, experts on fetal origins of disease think that children born with a higher-than-average birth weight went through a period of accelerated growth. During this time of excessive growth, it is possible that certain tissues, such as those that affected by leukemia and brain cancer, also undergo very rapid growth. Cells that undergo rapid growth and division are far more susceptible to the changes that may some day result in cancer.

The mechanism by which maternal hypertension increases leukemia risk is not yet identified. As with other factors, it could be that hypertension is simply a marker for another factor that is more directly related.

ASTHMA

Babies born too small or to mothers who smoked during pregnancy are more likely to develop asthma as young children. There is also some evidence that being born "late," or too much past the due date, might also increase the risk of developing asthma later in life.

Being poorly nourished at the end of pregnancy might be an important cause of asthma in early childhood. We can distinguish low birth weight that is caused by poor nourishment at the beginning of pregnancy from low birth weight that occurs because a woman is poorly nourished at the end by looking at the difference in babies' head circumference, or the size of the head at birth. Babies who are poorly nourished at the end of pregnancy tend to have a head circumference at birth that is disproportionately larger than their birth weight. This means that they probably sacrificed growth of certain body tissues to protect brain growth. One of the tissues that might have been compromised is the thymus gland. Normal thymus tissue is necessary to regulate allergic reactions and asthma.

Many people with asthma suffer from an underlying allergic condition as well. Allergists measure levels of an antibody called immunoglobulin E (IgE); they typically find that people with allergies have higher-than-normal levels of IgE. People who have high IgE levels as adults are far more likely to have been born past their due date.

There are three preventive steps you can take to reduce your child's chances of developing asthma. First, you can make certain you have excellent prenatal care. When an obstetrician or nurse midwife manages your pregnancy carefully, you are less likely to deliver your baby later than is healthy (being a few days past term should not be of concern). Second, stop smoking—for your own well-being as well as for your child's. Third, follow our dietary guidelines, which can help you gain just the right amount of weight and also help you and baby harvest all essential nutrients.

SCHIZOPHRENIA

Scientists have found that the constellation of disordered thinking called schizophrenia more often occurs in babies born to mothers who are poorly nourished during pregnancy; the chance increases even more when nutritional intake is low during the first trimester.

The brain and spinal cord is a very complex set of tissues and chemicals, all working together to allow us to perform all of our life functions, each and every day. Because the brain and spinal column develop so very early after conception—they are completely formed just 4 weeks after sperm meets egg—it is easy to understand why a lack of nutrition early on could adversely impact brain development. Indeed, a considerable amount of research has been done to try to understand why poor nutrition early in pregnancy can cause schizophrenia.

As we introduce this research, we'd like to make note of one more related factor. Prenatal experts have confirmed that a deficiency of folic acid, a B vitamin, is a significant cause of spina bifida and other neural tube defects (defects of the spinal column). As we said above, the brain and spinal column are all closely related. As it turns out, researchers have evidence that a folic acid deficiency may also contribute to schizophrenia.

Dr. Ezra Susser's research team, which has delved deeply into the prenatal environment–schizophrenia connection, has found several ways in which poor nutrition impacts the complex brain system. For one, poor nutrition prevents the proper development of the neurotransmitter system in the brain, which is a series of brain chemicals that relay messages from the brain to tissues and back again. Although it is important for mom and baby to get enough of all nutrients, a lack of protein in particular is thought to severely impact the development of the neurotransmitter system.

Poor nutrition is also thought to prevent a part of the brain called the hippocampus from developing optimally. The hippocampus is one of the emotion centers of the brain. In people who have schizophrenia, the hippocampus does not function properly, potentially because it was not well nourished during the time it was supposed to grow in utero.

PUTTING IT ALL INTO PERSPECTIVE

It may seem almost overwhelming to know that the nutrition and health habits you follow during pregnancy can have such a profound and long-lasting effect on the baby you are carrying or are about to carry. But let's turn this around into the beneficial knowledge it is: You may be able to positively impact your child-to-be's future health. You can make a contribution to provide your baby with the optimal environment in the womb that will favorably affect the rest of his or her life.

Don't worry if you are already into your pregnancy or if you have had other children. No matter where you are in your pregnancy, you can have that positive impact. Follow a healthy nutrition diet throughout your days in waiting like our Optimal Pregnancy Diet (see chapters that follow). Rather than focusing on "preventing" one complication or another, we recommend that you concentrate on taking good care of yourself during the full course of your pregnancy, part of which includes eating the optimal number of calories, protein, and nutrients each day. Doing so can help your baby grow optimally and perhaps minimize the chances that your child will develop high blood pressure, high cholesterol levels, and other chronic diseases later in his or her adult life.

I also want to remind you, though, that your contribution to your child's health isn't finished at birth. Nutrition during childhood and adolescence is of great relevance. Unfortunately, the diet of our children and adolescents leaves much to be desired today. Earn your reputation as a loving, knowledgeable, and yes, sometimes nagging mother and encourage your children—from the first days they begin to eat solid food—to eat nourishing food.

As he or she becomes an adult, your future child's health will also be very dependent on other factors such as maintaining a healthy body weight, exercising, getting enough sleep, and reducing stress. As a mother, you can instill healthy behavior by your own good example. Chapter Eleven will provide general guidelines on just how to do this.

In the next chapter, I'll introduce the goals and objectives that enable you to maximize nutrition in each stage of your pregnancy—and in the months preceding your pregnancy if you are still in the planning stage. Read on and learn how to achieve the best (and tastiest!) nutrition for you and your growing baby. As you might have guessed by now, we call this the Optimal Pregnancy Diet.

CHAPTER THREE

Goals, Objectives, and Calories . . . Calories . . . Calories

The Optimal Pregnancy Diet

The first two chapters of *The Gift of Health* have discussed the theory behind the new research into the fetal origins of disease. However, if you are already, or are planning to become, pregnant, I'm sure you're very eager to find out more about the Optimal Pregnancy Diet, which maximizes your chance of having a healthy baby who grows up to be a healthy adult. This chapter will expand on the goals and objectives of this new diet, from calorie levels and weight gain to the nutrients most important to your developing baby. These discussions lead into Chapter Four, which provides an essential overview of the diet, explaining how to use the meal plans and recipes we provide, how to develop your own meal plans, and how to adjust them to ensure you meet your weight gain goals.

For now, let's get into the specifics: what nutrients you need and, just as significant—perhaps even more so—the calories you need. Both of these factors are quintessentially important to your developing baby.

The three goals of our Optimal Pregnancy Diet are

- To prevent undernutrition in the first and third trimesters
- To prevent overnutrition in the second and third trimesters
- To maximize the notable nutrients during pregnancy: protein, vitamin B$_6$, folic acid, calcium, iron, zinc

Let's take a look at each of these in more detail.

To Prevent Undernutrition in the
First and Third Trimesters

It may seem odd to even talk about undernutrition in developed countries, where the general concern is about excesses—taking in too many calories, too much fat, too much sugar. Indeed, many women find themselves constantly battling with calories and trying to shave off a few here and there. But in the first and third trimesters of pregnancy, women often have a difficult time taking in enough calories—for quite different reasons in each trimester.

In the *first* trimester, women are often queasy (to say the least!) and thus may feel like avoiding food at all costs. Kris Napier, the dietitian who wrote this book with me, remembers going up to the second-floor bedroom most nights during the first trimester, taking the screen out, and sticking her head out of the window for some fresh air while her husband ate dinner! Getting enough calories can be exceptionally difficult during this time, especially calories with the right composition of nutrients.

In the *third* trimester, I can sum it all up in one word: *stuffed*. Women simply feel stuffed all the time. The rapidly growing baby pushes the stomach up into a little corner near the lungs, which also creates a feeling of breathlessness. This, too, makes getting the optimal number of calories difficult, especially calories that contain the appropriate amounts of nutrients.

Although I included the information in Chapters One and Two about the possible effects of taking in too few calories, let me just briefly review them here.

During the first trimester, taking in enough calories (and all the essential nutrients, as you'll read below) is critically important to ensuring optimal development of all the baby's organs and the placenta. Too few calories at this time, for example, can result in a smaller-than-normal liver, which can affect the ability to filter out excess cholesterol and other substances as an adult. Getting a scant number of calories may also cause an unborn child's metabolism to become what scientists call thrifty. This means that the body is stimulated to conserve and store calories whenever possible, to try to build up fat reserves in case of times of famine or hunger. As you can imagine, this can lead to a tendency to be overweight as an adult.

Equally as important, optimal nutrition during the first trimester is essential for developing a healthy placenta. Think of the placenta as the conduit that relays all nutrients and calories from mom to baby. If the placenta isn't fully developed, then all of the nutrients mom eats later in pregnancy will have a more difficult time getting to the developing fetus.

TO PREVENT OVERNUTRITION IN THE SECOND AND THIRD TRIMESTERS

True, undernutrition in the second trimester is also problematical. But this is quite unlikely—generally, women have the opposite problem! There is something magical about that transition from weeks 12 and 13 into week 14, the official start of the second trimester, when queasiness and nausea suddenly lift, leaving an incredibly healthy appetite. Truly, many women say they can mark the start of their second trimester simply because they woke up one day and weren't nauseated anymore!

This makes eating easier—lots easier. Sometimes, in fact, too easy! The hormonal changes that come with the second trimester often give women a tremendous sense of well-being. That terrible fatigue that accompanies the first trimester lifts as well, and energy levels are high. Those same hormonal changes may also send your appetite into overdrive. Although the cravings of pregnancy may seem like an old wives' tale, they really do happen. Pregnancy experts believe that they're probably hormonally based. Whatever the reason, they can be a real problem for some women—let's say *most* women! In fact, research reveals that about 85% of pregnant women experience cravings during this trimester. The trick is in learning to satisfy them without overspending the calorie budget.

Sometimes, women continue to have an overly healthy appetite in the third trimester. The reasons vary, but this could occur because the baby is lying in a position in the womb that doesn't crowd out the stomach. In other cases, a woman simply eats calorie-dense foods so frequently that she gains excessive weight.

Whatever the reasons, moms-to-be should avoid excess calorie intake in the second and third trimesters. Recommendations to gain as much weight as possible during pregnancy are not advisable for mother or child; gaining excessive weight in these trimesters may result in a baby that is heavier than the normal or average birth weight. Female babies born heavier may carry an increased risk of breast cancer as an adult. Both male and female babies may have an increased risk of becoming overweight (because more fat cells form).

MAXIMIZE THE NOTABLE NUTRIENTS

All nutrients that are essential to human beings are important during pregnancy. But there are certain nutrients that stand out ahead of all the others:

- Protein
- Vitamin B$_6$
- Folic acid
- Calcium
- Iron
- Zinc

Let's take a look at why they are so important. (A quick note about all of these notable nutrients: Not only are they particularly important during pregnancy but they are also often difficult to get enough of. That's why we've planned the meals and menus as we have, to make sure you can consume enough of all of them.) Following this discussion, you'll find two charts: One lists all nutrients required during pregnancy and how much you need. (I compare it with the amounts you need before pregnancy and also during breast-feeding, just for convenience). Another chart lists the foods that are particularly high in each notable nutrient.

Protein

Cells simply cannot be formed without protein, which provides the building blocks—amino acids—for growth to occur. But protein plays many more roles during pregnancy. A low protein intake may have serious implications that range from changes in the pancreas that predispose the baby to diabetes in later life, to inadequate development and function of the placenta. Researchers suspect that poor placental function due to a low protein intake may compromise the placenta's role in preventing harmful substances from passing from mother to baby. This includes cortisol, a stress hormone made by mom, which, if too much passes from the mother's to the baby's bloodstream, may affect the unborn baby's brain and cause it to be oversensitive to stress as an adult. The effect: a possible predisposition to high blood pressure many decades after birth.

Vitamin B$_6$

Also known as pyridoxine, this vitamin B$_6$ plays a couple of key roles during pregnancy. It is essential in the formation of the nervous system of the developing baby and for all rapidly dividing cells. (As you can imagine, your baby's cells are dividing rapidly, particularly in the earlier days of pregnancy.) In a quite different role, B$_6$ also helps Mom use the extra protein she requires during pregnancy. B$_6$ and protein provide a great example of how essential nutrients work together in the body. Even if Mom gets enough protein, she will be unable to use it without enough B$_6$.

Folic acid

Like zinc and vitamin B$_6$, folic acid is especially critical when cells divide rapidly. It serves as the shuttle bus that carries protein fragments, called amino acids, to areas under construction—especially the spinal column and palate. Because these needs are so important during the first days of pregnancy, when many women don't know they are pregnant, the U.S. government advises all women of childbearing age to consume at least 400 micrograms of folic acid daily, and some experts recommend 800 micrograms. The demand for folic acid remains high right through the last days of pregnancy, when it helps prevent premature birth, so a minimum of 600 micrograms per day is recommended during pregnancy. In one study, women who consumed less than 240 micrograms of folic acid during pregnancy doubled their risk of giving birth too early. Although we recommend that people get their nutrients from food rather than supplements, folic acid is one nutrient of which it's difficult to get sufficient amounts through diet alone, and thus a supplement (400 micrograms per day) is recommended.

Calcium

Critically important throughout a woman's life, calcium is even more important during pregnancy; it is a key factor in determining the strength of mother's and baby's bones. In another example of nutrients working together, calcium cannot work alone to build strong bones. We also require vitamin D, for example, which allows us to absorb the calcium from our diet, and magnesium, another key component in the structure of our bones. Other key bone-building nutrients include zinc, vitamin C, and vitamin K.

Iron

Pregnant or not, iron is one of the most difficult nutrients for women of childbearing age to get enough of. As a result, some women enter pregnancy anemic, a condition that can compromise the baby's normal development. So it's best to try to enter pregnancy with good iron stores. The best plan is to see a physician for a checkup before getting pregnant and then correct any existing anemia with a physician's help. During pregnancy, iron is important to both mother and baby. Not only does it prevent anemia in you (which can cause terrible fatigue) but it also helps your baby gain enough weight and helps prevent premature delivery. (Premature delivery is a real problem because babies born too soon may have difficulty breathing and can have other problems as well.)

One more important point: Iron cannot work alone to enable red blood cells to carry oxygen to the body's tissues and prevent anemia. The other blood-building nutrients include vitamin C, vitamin B_{12}, riboflavin, and copper.

Zinc

This mineral plays a key role in the very earliest days of pregnancy, when cells divide rapidly to form the tiny but recognizable shape of a baby. Like vitamin B_6, zinc is essential for the constant formation of the proteins that make up the different tissues of your baby. And like folic acid and iron, zinc also guards against giving birth too early.

Recommended Daily Intakes of Important Nutrients, Vitamins, and Minerals

	Woman, 19–24 Years	Woman, 25–50 Years	Pregnant Woman	Lactating Woman, First 6 Months	Lactating Woman, Second 6 Months
Protein (g)	46	50	60	65	62
Vitamin A (mcg RE)	700	700	770	1,300	1,200
Vitamin E (mg)	15	15	15	19	11
Vitamin K (mcg)	90	90	90	90	65
Vitamin C (mg)	75	75	85	120	90
Iron (mg)	18	18	27	9	15
Zinc (mg)	8	8	11	12	16

	Woman, 19–24 Years	Woman, 25–50 Years	Pregnant Woman	Lactating Woman, First 6 Months	Lactating Woman, Second 6 Months
Iodine (mcg)	150	150	220	290	200
Selenium (mcg)	55	55	60	70	75
Calcium (mg)	1,000	1,000	1,000	1,000	1,300
Phosphorus (mg)	700	700	700	700	700
Magnesium (mg)	310	320	350	310	320
Vitamin D (mcg)	5	5	5	5	5
Fluoride (mg)	3	3	3	3	3
Thiamin (mg)	1.1	1.1	1.4	1.4	1.5
Riboflavin (mg)	1.1	1.1	1.4	1.6	1.6
Niacin (mg)	14	14	18	17	17
Vitamin B_6 (mcg)	1.3	1.3	1.9	2.0	2.0
Folic acid (mcg)	400	400	600	500	500
Vitamin B_{12} (mcg)	2.4	2.4	2.6	2.8	2.8
Pantothenic acid (mg)	5	5	6	7	7
Biotin (mcg)	30	30	30	35	35
Choline (mg)	425	425	450	550	550

g = grams; mcg = micrograms; mcg RE = micrograms retinol equivalent; mg = milligrams
Information based on 2000 Dietary Reference Intakes and 1989 Recommended Dietary
Allowances, National Academy of Sciences.

Good Food Sources for the Notable Nutrients

Nutrient	Food Sources
Vitamin B_6	Whole-grain foods, meat, eggs, dried beans and peas, nuts, bananas, avocados
Calcium	Dairy foods, fortified orange juice, fortified soy milk, dark green leafy vegetables, dried beans and peas, nuts, salmon and sardines (canned with bones)
Folic acid	Dark green leafy vegetables, oranges, dried beans and peas, papaya, blueberries, raspberries, strawberries, asparagus, lima beans, fortified grain foods, pineapple
Iron	Meat, poultry, fish, dried beans and peas, whole-grain foods, dark green leafy vegetables, fortified breakfast cereal
Protein	Poultry, fish, dairy foods, meat, dried beans and peas, soy products
Zinc	Poultry, fish, whole-grain foods, meat, dried beans and peas, nuts, seeds, wheat germ, soy products

CALORIE MADNESS

All mothers-to-be are concerned about weight gain, striking that delicate balance between gaining too little and too much. And we've emphasized again and again the importance of avoiding under- or overnutrition with an appropriate calorie intake. So you're probably asking yourself: *How many calories do I need?* Bear in mind that no two expectant women have the same initial weight before pregnancy or at conception, nor do they have the same metabolic rate. Thus, no one calorie intake can be the optimum for all women trying to get pregnant or for all pregnant women. In addition, calorie requirements can change during pregnancy as you gain weight at a faster rate in the later trimesters (more about that a little later).

That's just one of the ways in which *The Gift of Health* is different from all other pregnancy books. We've provided you with

- A choice of three different calorie levels to follow before pregnancy, depending on whether you need to maintain, gain, or lose weight
- The option of two calorie levels for each of the three trimesters of pregnancy, based on your size, activity level, and appetite

Before we take a more detailed look at how to decide what level is right for you and your baby-to-be, I'd like to mention two additional points about where your calories come from. The first has to do with the proportion of your calories that come from protein and carbohydrates. Here's a quick nutrition lesson: You should know that the calories in your food are divided among three major sources—protein, carbohydrate, and fat. U.S. health officials recommend that we all get 50% to 60% of our calories from complex carbohydrates, 15% to 25% as protein, and 20% to 30% as fat. Dividing calories thusly is also a way to help you take in all the nutrients you need for good health and disease prevention. When you are pregnant, dividing your calories optimally has even greater dividends.

As you read in Chapter Two, British researchers led by Dr. Barker have shown that eating the optimal type of calories affects the weight of the placenta—which in turn impacts the baby's health. Moms who had too many carbohydrate calories and not enough protein calories in early pregnancy delivered both babies and placentas that were of lower weight than the healthy average. In late pregnancy, eating too little protein predisposed mothers to gave birth to lighter-than-average babies and placentas. This gives additional importance to the recommendations for intake of these nutrients given by the Food and Nutrition Board of the National Academy of Sciences. Rest assured, we have followed these recommendations in every one of our meal plans and do-it-yourself guidelines to ensure that you get just the right amount of all types of calories.

The other issue about calories is even more specific: It has to do with the type of fat calories you consume. There is preliminary evidence from animal studies that getting too many calories from polyunsaturated fatty acids may increase a female rat's offspring's risk of breast cancer. This is one of the reasons why we have designed all of our trimester optimal diets (and the prepregnancy optimal diet) with a preponderance of monounsaturated fats. (See "About Fats," page 79, to read about different types of fat.) Keep in mind, however, that this information about the type of fat consumed in pregnancy stems from research that is still at the laboratory animal stage. But monounsaturated fats are preferable for another reason: Getting a higher percentage of your fat calories from monounsaturated fats protects against atherosclerosis, or coronary artery disease.

PREPREGNANCY CALORIE LEVELS

We've designed highly nutritious "in training" meal plans at

- 1,700 calories
- 1,900 calories
- 2,100 calories

How do you decide which one to follow? Part of this is based on your prepregnancy weight and body mass index (BMI). Please refer to the chart on the next page.

FINDING YOUR BODY MASS INDEX

BMI is a tool health professionals use to determine whether a person's weight is appropriate for his or her height. It is based on a mathematical equation, however, so to make life simpler, we have provided the table on the next page with everyone's equation already calculated.

Simply find your height in feet and inches on the left-hand column, then find your weight in the top row. Move down and across until the columns intersect. That number is your BMI. A BMI between 20 and 25 indicates that you are a healthy weight for your height. Under 20 corresponds to being underweight, and over 25, to being overweight.

Body Mass Index* Calculator

Weight in Pounds

Height	90	100	110	120	130	140	150	160	170	180	190	200	210	220	230	240	250	260	270	280	290	300
4'6"	22	24	27	29	31	34	36	39	41	43	46	48	51	53	56	58	60	63	65	68	70	72
4'7"	21	23	26	28	30	33	35	37	40	42	44	47	49	51	54	56	58	61	63	65	68	70
4'8"	20	22	25	27	29	31	34	36	38	40	43	45	47	49	52	54	56	58	61	63	65	67
4'9"	20	22	24	26	28	30	33	35	37	39	41	43	46	48	50	52	54	56	59	61	63	65
4'10"	19	21	23	25	27	29	31	34	36	38	40	42	44	46	48	50	52	54	57	59	61	63
4'11"	18	20	22	24	26	28	30	32	34	36	38	40	42	44	46	48	51	53	55	57	59	61
5'0"	18	20	22	23	25	27	29	31	33	35	37	39	41	43	45	47	49	51	53	55	57	59
5'1"	17	19	21	23	25	27	28	30	32	34	36	38	40	42	44	45	47	49	51	53	55	57
5'2"	16	18	20	22	24	26	28	30	31	33	35	37	38	40	42	44	46	48	49	51	53	55
5'3"	16	18	20	21	23	25	27	29	31	32	34	36	38	39	41	43	44	46	48	50	51	53
5'4"	15	17	19	21	22	24	26	28	29	31	33	34	36	38	40	41	43	45	46	48	50	52
5'5"	15	17	18	20	22	23	25	27	28	30	32	33	35	37	38	40	42	43	45	47	48	50
5'6"	15	16	18	19	21	23	24	26	27	29	31	32	34	36	37	39	40	42	44	45	47	49
5'7"	14	16	17	19	20	22	23	25	27	28	30	31	33	34	36	38	39	41	42	44	45	47
5'8"	14	15	17	18	20	21	23	24	26	27	29	30	32	34	35	37	38	40	41	43	44	46
5'9"	13	15	16	18	19	21	22	24	25	27	28	30	31	33	34	35	37	38	40	41	43	44
5'10"	13	14	16	17	19	20	22	23	24	26	27	29	30	32	33	34	36	37	39	40	42	43
5'11"	13	14	15	17	18	20	21	22	24	25	27	28	29	31	32	34	35	36	38	39	41	42
6'0"	12	14	15	16	18	19	20	22	23	24	26	27	28	30	31	33	34	35	37	38	39	41
6'1"	12	13	15	16	17	18	20	21	22	24	25	26	28	29	30	32	33	34	36	37	38	40
6'2"	12	13	14	15	17	18	19	21	22	23	24	26	27	28	30	31	32	33	35	36	37	39
6'3"	11	12	14	15	16	18	19	20	21	23	24	25	26	28	29	30	31	33	34	35	36	38
6'4"	11	12	13	15	16	17	18	20	21	22	23	24	26	27	28	29	30	32	33	34	35	37
6'5"	11	12	13	14	15	16	18	19	20	21	23	24	25	26	27	29	30	31	32	33	34	36
6'6"	10	12	13	14	15	16	17	19	20	21	22	23	24	25	27	28	29	30	31	32	34	35

*Body mass index = weight in kilograms divided by height in meters squared.

To have the healthiest pregnancy, you should start it at a weight that is within your healthy weight range. In terms of BMI, you should start your pregnancy being between 20 and 25 if possible. As odd as it seems, it is just as undesirable to be underweight as to be overweight before your pregnancy. Here's why:

- When a woman is underweight before pregnancy, her infant has a greater chance of being underweight at birth.
- When a woman is overweight, she is at considerably increased risk of developing hypertension (elevated blood pressure) and diabetes during pregnancy and of having to have a cesarian section.

If you are below your healthy weight or have a BMI under 20, then please try to gain weight to bring yourself into this range. Unfortunately, gaining weight healthily is not as easy as adding a couple of candy bars or a hot fudge sundae to your daily eating plan. Such foods do contain plenty of calories, but they are also empty-calorie foods, virtually devoid of vitamins and minerals. Instead, please use the 2,100-calorie meal plan provided in Chapter Five. If you still aren't gaining, then please add in foods by 100-calorie increments from the tables in the section in Chapter Four entitled "What If I'm Not Gaining Weight?" on pages 97 through 98.

If you are already within your healthy weight range, you should follow one of the three calorie levels listed with the goal of maintaining your weight within this range until you become pregnant. Which calorie level you need will vary, depending on your height, frame size, and activity level. For the most part, though, women of childbearing age generally maintain their weight with about 1,900 calories a day. I suggest you start at this level and either increase or decrease your level if your weight changes.

Finally, if you are overweight, try to lose weight before your pregnancy begins—but do so ever so slowly. Please don't try to lose more than 2 pounds per week. Losing rapidly has several pitfalls. First, you will drain your body of nutrients you will need during those earliest days of pregnancy when you might not even know you are pregnant. Second, you may lose too much muscle mass. Finally, your body won't have a chance to adjust to your new weight and metabolism. You may not lose enough to reach your healthy weight range, but take heart, every pound lost (at a prudent, slow rate) means a healthier pregnancy.

So if you do need to lose weight, please start at 1,700 calories and exercise regularly so that the weight you lose is from your fat stores rather than from your muscles. If you find that you're not losing, you can either increase your activity (this is preferable; just add a daily 20- to 30-minute brisk walk) or decrease your calories by 100. To decrease calories and maintain the nutrition that preloads your cells for the healthiest pregnancy possible, please drop one of the grain food servings from your meal plan. You can do this by dropping one entire serving from one meal or snack, or by eliminating half a serving from one menu item and half from another. (You can find out more about grain food serving sizes in the table "Grain Gallery" on page 86.)

If you are trying to lose a few pounds, we would like you to take a multivitamin and mineral supplement that supplies 100% of the Dietary Reference Intake (DRI) for women.

THE PREGNANCY 300

As odd as it seems, you need just 300 extra calories each day of your pregnancy; in fact, most women don't even need the extra 300 during the first trimester. In food terms, 300 calories is equivalent to two 8-ounce glasses of skim milk, one whole-grain serving, one fruit serving, and one vegetable serving. (See Chapter Four for definitions of these servings.) With all of the protein, vitamins, and minerals needed for your baby's development coming from just these few extra calories, you can see why it is so important to choose nutrient-dense foods each day and to eliminate the junk food.

To assist every woman in finding the right calorie level for herself during the various stages of her pregnancy, I have begun by providing two calorie levels in each of the pregnancy trimester meal plans, 1,900 and 2,200 calories. To aid in fine-tuning calorie levels for individual requirements, there are guidelines (found in Chapter Four) for adding or subtracting calories in 100-calorie increments to reach the exact intake needed to gain weight at the required rate. As everyone's requirements and metabolism are different, you may need to do a little experimenting.

I suggest that you follow the general guidelines below to find the right calorie level for you. (More detailed guidelines are found in the chapters that discuss the individual trimesters.)

In Trimester 1

Begin at the 1,900-calorie level, unless you required a higher calorie level to maintain your weight before pregnancy. In the latter case, begin at that higher calorie level. If your weight gain is slower than 1 pound every 2 to 4 weeks, increase your intake by one to three 100-calorie snacks daily, using the snack lists given in Chapter Four (page 97). (So that you add a variety of extra nutrients with your extra calories, I recommend that you add snacks from different food groups rather than just concentrating on the one type of food.) If your weight gain is faster, then reduce your intake by 100 calories per day, using the snack list. If you are still gaining weight too quickly, you may even need to drop a further 100 to 200 calories daily. I'd recommend that you reduce your intake of grain foods, nut and seeds, or fruit, rather than the valuable protein foods or dairy foods. And to ensure you aren't missing out on any nutrients, I'd recommend you ask your health care provider about a multivitamin and mineral supplement.

In Trimesters 2 and 3

This is where those extra 300 calories, or the pregnancy 300, as I call them, come in. If you maintained your prepregnant weight at around 1,900 calories, then 2,200 is a good target for each day of your second and third trimesters. If you are gaining too quickly or too slowly, then you can simply adjust your intake as outlined for the first trimester.

As I mentioned, this plan may require some fine-tuning to get the calorie levels just right for you and your baby, and you may need to adjust them further as your metabolism changes and your baby grows, but that is really the beauty of the Optimal Pregnancy Diet—it allows *you* to devise the best diet for *your* special needs.

TIPPING THE SCALES: A POUND-BY-POUND GUIDE

Often, one of the first questions women ask about pregnancy is how much weight they should gain. Again, as every woman begins pregnancy at a different weight and has a different metabolic rate, there is no exact answer for everyone. The general guideline, for women who begin pregnancy within their healthy weight range, is a total of 25 to 35 pounds. Ideally, it would be put on at a rate of

- 1 pound every 2 to 4 weeks during the first trimester (3 to 6 pounds total during this trimester) when your baby is developing rapidly but not growing very large

- 1 pound per week in the second and third trimesters (about 12 or 13 pounds during each trimester) when your baby is growing more rapidly

If, when you become pregnant, your weight is above or below your healthy weight range, discuss your recommended rate of weight gain with your obstetrician—it may vary slightly from the rates given above.

Will I Retain the Weight I Gain?

Scientific studies have shown that weight gained during the second and third trimesters is easily lost, whereas excess weight gained during the first trimester is often retained. Although more women have trouble gaining weight in the first trimester rather than gain too much, this does provide an added incentive to gain at an appropriate rate.

The next question on women's minds, given the total weight gained during pregnancy and the fact that babies weigh only 7 or 8 pounds, is where all those extra pounds are going. As you'll see from "Where Does

---

Where Does the Extra Weight Go?

A normal weight gain during your 9-month pregnancy is 25 to 35 pounds even though babies generally weigh only 7 or 8 pounds at birth. For a 28-pound weight gain during pregnancy, the extra weight distributes as follows:

Location	Weight (pounds)
Fetus	7.5
Placenta	1.5
Amniotic fluid	2.0
Uterus	2.0
Breasts	1.0
Blood	3.0
Water	3.5
Fat	7.5

From the Olson Center for Women's Health, University of Nebraska Medical Center.

the Extra Weight Go?" on the previous page, it goes into the placenta, the amniotic fluid, and many other parts of mom's body—we even need extra blood when we are pregnant! So you can see that it is imperative that we eat as well as possible every day, not just for the growth of our baby but also for our own bodies to prepare for and develop during the pregnancy.

We've learned a lot about the Optimal Pregnancy Diet's objectives in this chapter, and the importance of choosing an appropriate calorie level. Now let's move on to Chapter Four, which gets down to the nuts and bolts of how to use the diet.

CHAPTER FOUR

🍎

The Don't-Miss-It Overview

The Optimal Pregnancy Diet

To achieve the three goals of our Optimal Pregnancy Diet—to prevent undernutrition in the first and third trimesters, to prevent excessive weight gain in the second and third trimesters, and to maximize the notable nutrients every day of your pregnancy—you need to understand how the diet works and how it's organized. We have developed an organizational system that is extremely simple to understand and even easier to implement.

That's what this Don't-Miss-It Overview is all about. In a nutshell, our Optimal Pregnancy Diet is divided into *four* trimesters. Although this may seem odd at first, you'll soon appreciate that it makes perfect sense. In addition to the three trimesters you already know about, we've added a fourth: the few months before you become pregnant. This is a time for you to gear up your body to be in the greatest health possible, to withstand the physical marathon that is pregnancy. You might like to think of this as we do . . . as the training trimester. If you are not yet pregnant and still thinking about conceiving, then take a close look at Chapter Five and learn about how to get your body in shape for the long race.

THE OPTIMAL PREGNANCY DIET: A GENERAL DESCRIPTION

During each trimester of pregnancy, your body undergoes different types of changes. As a result, *you* feel quite different. In addition, the baby inside of you undergoes quite different "construction projects" in each trimester. Because distinct things happen to you and to baby in each of these 3-month segments, the demands on your body, nutritionally speaking, are quite different.

To address this, we've arranged our diet trimester by trimester so that it can meet all of these unique needs. This way, too, you can easily jump in wherever you are in your pregnancy. Just for the record, Chapter Five concerns prepregnancy, Chapter Six is for the first trimester, Chapter Seven the second trimester, and Chapter Eight details nutritional needs and menus for the third trimester.

How Each Chapter Is Organized

Each of these trimester chapters first provides an overview of what is happening in both your body and your baby's body, and then, in a section entitled "Nutrition Priorities," discusses how nutrition needs change during each one. Here, too, we'll outline why each trimester's diet differs from the others. You'll learn, for example, why folic acid is so critically important in the first trimester and why it surfaces again in the third trimester as a notable nutrient—but for quite a different reason.

After "Nutrition Priorities," you'll find 2 weeks' worth of meal plans for each different calorie level. As you read in Chapter Three, in the section entitled "Calorie Madness," we've provided you with three calorie levels to choose from in the prepregnancy "training trimester," and two calorie levels for each of the trimesters of pregnancy. In each of the next four chapters, we'll reiterate how you can decide which calorie level is best for you. We'll also teach you how to create additional nutritious meal plans on your own.

More About Our Meal Plans

Our meal plans are designed to translate your nutritional priorities during each trimester into food you can eat every day. To really simplify your life, we've converted the nutrients you need into real foods, real recipes, and real all-day meal plans. Yes, that means you don't have to do any planning if you don't want to!

Our meal plans are even more of a sanity-saver for a very important reason: Within each trimester's menus and within each calorie level, every breakfast has the same number of calories as every other breakfast for those 2 weeks' worth of menus. This means that you can exchange any breakfast within those 14 days for any other breakfast. The same is true for each lunch and each dinner within that menu.

As you have already guessed, this means that you can mix and match the breakfasts, lunches, and dinners to come up with 2,744 possible different combinations. That should be enough to get you through your pregnancy! However, if you want even more variety, we teach you how to design your own meal plans.

First, we convert your requirements into the appropriate number of servings from each food group. (At the end of this chapter, we've detailed serving sizes so that you know exactly what you need to eat if you choose to plan your meals by food groups.) Next, we divide those servings between meals and snacks, just a little differently to answer the needs of your changing body each trimester.

Food Preferences

Everybody has different dietary preferences. Some women love pasta, others can't live without chocolate. We cannot provide meal plans that hit everybody's taste buds alike. Therefore, we have given you the option to mix and choose among the meal options.

Also, we want you to enjoy the food. While we advocate to consume as many vegetables, fruits, and whole grain products as possible, we realize that for many of you it would be difficult to give up meat, pasta, and margarine altogether. Thus we have compromised to offer on average two vegetarian, two fish, and two meat dinners per week. This provides a healthy balance. If you wish to increase on the vegetarian and fish dinners and cut out the meat feel free to do so.

If you can replace pasta with whole grain pasta (which may not be available everywhere) or any other whole grain we encourage you to do so as well. Enjoy!

Troubleshooting

We know there will still be some lingering questions each trimester—questions that may be unique to those three months. So, we've added a "Troubleshooting" section to each chapter—and tried to think of everything you might want to know.

ABOUT THE OPTIMAL FOODS IN THE
OPTIMAL PREGNANCY DIET

We don't want you to waste a single calorie during your days in waiting. That is, we want to make sure that every food you eat will help your baby grow optimally and that you meet those demands with the minimum amount of stress on your system. Of course, demand is greatest for those notable nutrients we discussed in Chapter Three: protein, folic acid, vitamin B_6, calcium, iron, and zinc.

In nutrition language, we say that some foods are nutrient-dense. These foods have loads of nutrients relative to the calories they provide. The opposite of a nutrient-dense food is an empty-calorie food. I'm sure you've heard that term before! Examples of empty-calorie foods include potato chips, soda, candy bars, and many other snack foods.

We explain this because we have used many nutrient-dense foods over and over again, particularly those that are rich in the very important, but often hard to come by, notable nutrients. Because these foods are so valuable, we call them optimal pregnancy foods. So that you'll understand why these certain foods crop up again and again, we've included a brief summary of them here.

The Greens

There are salad greens . . . and then there are salad greens. If ever there were one food to fuss over choosing in the produce aisle, it would be salad greens. Greens are an important source—*the most* important source—of folic acid, one of the notable nutrients of pregnancy. Different greens are also high in several minerals that you and your baby need, including the notable nutrients calcium and iron. Here, we've listed some of the greens that we'd like you to learn to use, and a little description of each. As you'll see in the table on page 77, different greens are rich in different vitamins and minerals, which is why you'll find a great variety of them used in our meal plans. As they also have different flavors, try them all to see which you enjoy the most.

- *Arugula:* This leafy salad green has a delicious and subtle peppery mustard flavor. It is one of the few nonfish foods that are very high in omega-3 fatty acids, a type of fat that may help prevent heart disease and inflammation.

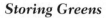

Storing Greens

When you buy fresh greens, store them unwashed in a plastic bag in the refrigerator crisper. Tear off what you will use for any particular meal or snack and wash just before you use it. Rinse by running cold water over the leaves or by soaking loose leaves in the sink or in a large bowl of cool water. (If leaves are muddy or particularly dirty, wash them two or three times.) Lay out the washed leaves on clean cotton dishtowels or paper towels, allowing excess water to drain off, or dry them in a salad spinner.

- *Dandelion greens:* These are the green, jagged leaves of the yellow-flowered weed. The flavor is tangy and somewhat bitter. Leaves should be bright green, not yellow.
- *Iceberg lettuce:* Also called crisphead lettuce, it comes in a pale green head of tightly packed leaves. Iceberg is an old favorite and adds crispy texture to salads. Try to mix this lettuce in with some darker greens to get a good mix of nutrients.
- *Mesclun greens:* Usually found in a supermarket as salad mix, it is just that—a mix of different, small salad greens. It usually includes arugula, dandelion, frisee, mizuma, oak leaf, mache, radicchio, and sorrel—all greens rich in nutrients.
- *Mustard greens:* These leaves of the mustard plant are dark green with a peppery, pungent flavor. They are best enjoyed cooked, such as in soups and stews, but many people eat them raw.
- *Romaine lettuce:* Also called cos lettuce, romaine has long, leafy leaves with dark green tips that fade into bright green and then white bottoms. The midrib is crisp, and the outer leaves are much softer. Try to choose the darkest green romaine you can, which helps you harvest loads more folic acid and minerals.
- *Spinach:* This nutritionally packed veggie has dark green leaves that are usually smooth, depending on the variety. Enjoy it *very* fresh, but don't hesitate to have frozen on hand for a quick meal. It's a green that is also a great cooked vegetable.
- *Watercress:* This member of the mustard family gets its name from the watery ground where it grows. Its leaves are small and dark green with a wonderfully unique flavor that has just a hint of pepper.

Green Vitamins and Minerals

Greens (2 Cups Raw)	Vitamin A (Amount/% Pregnancy RDA)	Vitamin E (Amount/% Pregnancy RDA)	Vitamin C (Amount/% Pregnancy RDA)	Vitamin K (Amount/% Pregnancy RDA)	Folic acid (Amount/% Pregnancy RDA)	Calcium (Amount/% Pregnancy RDA)
Arugula	94.80 RE/12%	0.17 mg/2%	6.0 mg/9%	148 mcg/255%	38.80 mg/10%	64.0 mg/5%
Dandelion greens	1,540 RE/193%	2.75 mg/28%	38.50 mg/55%	444 mcg/765%	29.92 mcg/7%	205.7 mg/17%
Iceberg lettuce	36.30 RE/5%	0.31 mg/3%	4.29 mg/6%	0.19 mcg/0%	61.60 mcg/15%	20.90 mg/2%
Mesclun greens	510.10 RE/54%	1.47 mg/15%	16.94 mg/24%	208 mcg/358%	58.28 mcg/15%	86.08 mg/7%
Mustard greens	593.60 RE/74%	2.25 mg/23%	78.40 mg/112%	190.40 mcg/328%	209.44 mcg/52%	115.36 mg/10%
Romaine lettuce	291.2 RE/36%	0.49 mg/5%	26.88 mg/38%	0.22 mcg/0%	152.32 mcg/38%	40.32 mg/3%
Spinach	403.2 RE/50%	1.13 mg/11%	16.86 mg/24%	240.00 mcg/413%	116.4 mcg/29%	59.40 mg/5%
Watercress	319.6 RE/40%	0.68 mg/7%	6.0 mg/9%	170 mcg/293%	38.80 mcg/10%	64.0 mg/5%

mcg = microgram(s); mg = milligram(s); RE = retinol equivalent.

Optimal Oil—Olive, That Is!—and Margarine

You'll notice that olive oil is just about the only added fat you'll find in our menus. This is because olive oil is good for you—in the right, healthy amounts it is the best type of fat to use when you must use fat. It is high in monounsaturated fat, which is probably the healthiest of fats—in moderation. Olive oil is the primary source of fat in Southern European populations who have the world's highest longevity. But since olive oil is low in some other essential fatty acids, linolenic and linoleic, we need to get these elsewhere. Good sources are soybeans, walnuts, flaxseed and flaxseed oil, canola oil, and fish, especially salmon, mackerel, tuna, and trout. Kris has used two different types or grades of olive oil, depending on the foods it is paired with or the recipe it's in: light or virgin olive oil. Virgin, or the more strongly flavored and darkly colored extra-virgin, oil has a much more powerful flavor that is used when you want to taste the oil, such as a salad dressing. Try to get the cold-pressed variety—it has even more nutrients. Light, as the name implies, is much milder in flavor, and is suitable for recipes when you don't want to taste it in the food, such as cooking desserts. See the table "Virgin or Light: What's Right?" for more guidelines. Light olive oil also works better for sautéing because it doesn't burn as easily as extra-virgin.

Virgin or Light: What's Right?

	Use Virgin or Extra-Virgin Olive Oil	*Use Light or Extra-Light Olive Oil*
Dipping bread	√	
Bruschetta	√	
Salad dressing	√	√
Marinating grilled vegetables (such as eggplant, peppers, portobello mushrooms)	√	
Strongly flavored pasta sauces	√	
Creamy pasta sauces		√
General frying and sautéing (use light for more delicately flavored foods; if frying at very high temperatures, use light)		√
Sweet foods		√

A word about margarine: Margarine is one of those foods that many of us like on our toast, but it is better to try to leave it out of your meal plan. Here's why. Most versions contain a lot of *trans*-fatty acids, also called *trans*-fats, substances that are produced when margarines are made by hardening liquid oils. *Trans*-fatty acids are very bad for the heart (see "About Fats" below). We're going to help you find a happy medium in two ways. First, as mentioned above, we've used olive oil in most recipes where you would usually use margarine. Second, following are guidelines for how to choose a

---

About Fats

Nature constructs several types of fat. Although they all have the same number of calories per gram (9) and are quite similar in structure, they each behave differently in the body. The three main types of fat are saturated, monounsaturated, and polyunsaturated fats.

Saturated fats are one of the most important factors responsible for raising blood cholesterol levels. This type of fat is thought to prohibit the liver from filtering out bad cholesterol from the bloodstream, thus raising the risk of heart disease. Saturated fat is found in animal products such as meat and dairy foods (except fat-free dairy) and in many processed foods such as bakery products and high-fat fast food and snack foods. The only plant foods that contain saturated fats are coconut, coconut oil, and palm oil.

Polyunsaturated fats, or polys, are generally good fats. Like the optimal fat type, monounsaturated, polys lower blood cholesterol when substituted for saturated fats. Polys seem to be beneficial for the prevention of coronary heart desease and diabetes. Polys are found in many vegetable oils, including sunflower, safflower, corn, and soybean, and in some types of nuts, especially walnuts. An especially valuable type of polyunsaturated fat called omega-3 is found in fish, especially those that come from cold waters, such as mackerel and salmon.

Monounsaturated fat is the optimal type of fat to include in your diet. The best source for it is olive oil, followed by canola oil,

(continued)

About Fats (continued)

peanut oil, and avocados. Nuts are also good sources of monoun-saturated fats.

Trans-fats are not naturally occurring fats. They are the by-products of a chemical process. When liquid vegetable oils are hardened to produce solid fats such as margarine or vegetable shortening, the chemical configuration of those fats change and *trans*-fats are produced. Watch out for the terms *hydrogenated* and, in particular, *partially hydrogenated,* which you will find on the ingredient label of many processed foods, especially many cookies and cakes. *Trans*-fats have been found to clog our arteries even worse than saturated fats do and therefore raise the risk of a heart attack.

So why do food manufacturers put these fats into our foods if they are so bad for us? Because (partially) hydrogenated fats increase the shelf life of foods, which, of course, is a great benefit to the industry. But not to our arteries.

Practically speaking, the best advice is to avoid saturated and, in particular, *trans*-fats as best you can in your diet and replace them whenever possible with monounsaturated fats.

---

margarine if you must use one. Rather than use brand names, which can change, we're listing what you should look for on the label.

First, try to find a margarine that is made mainly with monounsaturated fats, canola, or preferably olive oil. Then look for information on *trans*-fats. Just because a label says "all-vegetable margarine" or "saturated fat free" or "part of a heart-healthy diet" doesn't mean it is *trans*-fat free. What you should look for on the label are any of the following phrases:

- 0 *trans*-fats
- *trans*-fat free
- 0 grams *trans*-fat
- No *trans*-fatty acids

So what about butter, you will ask. For years, recommendations have been going back and forth about which is worse, butter or margarine.

Butter has relatively little *trans*-fat but, of course, is loaded with saturated fat. Butter is probably less bad than a margarine full of *trans*-fat, but a *trans*-fat–free margarine is probably preferable.

The Nuts and Seeds

Yes, you'll be seeing nuts and seeds quite regularly in our meal plans—but just certain ones. Let me explain why we want you to includes nuts and seeds, and then the reason for focusing on specific ones. Also, make sure you read our note about dry-roasted versus oil-roasted nuts below.

Dry-Roasted Versus Oil-Roasted Nuts

Make an effort to choose dry-roasted instead of oil-roasted nuts. There are a number of reasons why:

- **Oil-roasted nuts have added oils and thus more calories than dry-roasted.**
- **The oil used to roast nuts often either is saturated or contains *trans*-fatty acids.**
- **Oil-roasted nuts are more often heavily salted.**

Nuts and seeds are a great—in fact, phenomenal—source of many minerals that most Americans usually get from eating meat. Some of these minerals are the notable nutrients zinc, selenium, magnesium, copper, and manganese. Why get minerals from nuts and seeds instead of from meat? For one, nuts and seeds are plant-based foods, or nonanimal foods, and the great majority of vegetable foods have a more favorable fat profile than do animal foods—in other words, they are lower in saturated fat, and the ones we have chosen are high in monounsaturated fats.

That said, we are quick to add that some nuts didn't do so well when Mother Nature was planning their fat profile. That's why we'd like you to focus on including certain nuts and seeds over others. The ones with the best fat profile, and that you'll see frequently in our menus, are

- *Almonds:* Sweet almonds, the type available in the United States, are known for their delicate flavor. Almonds are packed with nutritional value and available in several different forms.

- *Hazelnuts:* Also called filberts, hazelnuts are wild nuts common in Europe. In the United States they are grown mainly in Oregon and Washington. Hazelnuts grow on trees in clusters. They have a sweet and rich flavor with a bitter brown covering that is removed before eating. They can be added to salads, main dishes, and desserts to add flavor and texture.
- *Macadamia nuts:* These delicious nuts are native to Australia but grown mostly in Hawaii. Once cracked from their hard brown shell, the kernel is eaten raw or roasted, or it can be pressed to yield a delicious cooking oil.
- *Peanuts:* Also called ground nuts, earth nuts, or goober peas, these nuts, which are actually legumes, are covered in a brown, papery skin and contained in a tan-colored netted shell or pod. Peanuts are sold both shelled and unshelled. Many are roasted and/or salted. The two most common varieties are Spanish peanuts and Virginia peanuts.
- *Pumpkin seeds:* Whoever thought this seed that so many people throw away when carving their pumpkins would be such a nutritional powerhouse? It's a great source of zinc and copper.
- *Soy nuts:* Like peanuts, soy nuts are really a legume; you might also see them called permut nuts. They are the roasted version of the soybean. You'll see that soy nuts are much lower in fat than other nuts. Soy nuts are also high in folic acid, that so-essential pregnancy nutrient.
- *Sunflower seeds:* The hulled little seed of the sunflower plant is packed full of vitamin B_6 and folic acid, two of the notable nutrients. It's also quite high in several other vitamins and minerals. Alone or as a topper for salad, yogurt, or cereal, sunflower seeds add a wonderful crunch.
- *Walnuts:* Of the two varieties, English and black, the English walnuts are the most commonly used. Walnuts generally come in three sizes when in the shell: baby, medium, and large. Because their fat turns bad quickly, they must be stored in a container in the refrigerator and should be eaten fairly quickly.

Nutrients in a Nutshell

Nut	Calories per Ounce	% Saturated Fat	% Monounsaturated Fat	% Polyunsaturated Fat	Rich in These Nutrients
Almonds	166.4	9.9%	67.6%	22.5%	Riboflavin, niacin, vitamin E, copper, magnesium, manganese
Hazelnuts	183	6%	61%	11%	Vitamin B$_6$, biotin, folic acid, vitamin E, copper, magnesium, manganese, and zinc
Macadamias	199.02	15.3%	82.4%	2.3%	Magnesium
Peanuts	165.9	14.9%	52.2%	32.9%	Niacin, copper, magnesium, manganese, phosphorus, zinc
Soy nuts	128.4	15.8%	23.7%	60.5%	Folic acid, copper, magnesium, manganese, selenium, zinc
Walnuts	172.1	6.8%	23.3%	69.9%	Copper, magnesium, manganese, selenium

The Soy Products

The tiny, ancient soybean contains significant amounts of all the notable nutrients we keep mentioning: folic acid, zinc, calcium, iron, vitamin B$_6$, and protein, as well as many other nutrients. In addition, it is almost void of saturated fat and low in total fat overall. Below is a brief explanation of the various soy products and a table with nutritional information.

- *Soymilk:* This milky liquid is an alternative to cow's milk because it is a nondairy product. Be sure to purchase fortified, lower-fat soymilk. It also comes in flavors such as chocolate and vanilla.

Soy Statistics

Soy Product	Calories	Protein	Fat	Rich in These Nutrients
Soy milk (1 cup)	130	10 g	4 g	Protein, vitamin A, thiamin, vitamin B_{12}, vitamin E, calcium, magnesium, phosphorus, potassium
Soy nuts (½ cup)	190.26	15.54 g	10.08 g	Folic acid, copper, magnesium, manganese, phosphorus, potassium, zinc
Tempeh (3 oz.)	169.25	16.16 g	6.53 g	Niacin, vitamin B_6, vitamin B_{12}, copper, magnesium, manganese, phosphorus, zinc, selenium
TVP (2 oz.)	153.09	30.05 g	0.57 g	Thiamin, riboflavin, niacin, vitamin B_6, vitamin B_{12}, folic acid, pantothenic acid, calcium, copper, iron, magnesium, manganese, phosphorus, zinc
Light tofu (3 oz.)	31.30	5.26 g	0.68 g	Calcium, copper, iron, magnesium, phosphorus, zinc

g = gram(s); oz. = ounce(s); TVP = textured vegetable protein.

- *Soy nuts:* See above, under "The Nuts and Seeds."
- *Tempeh (also called tempe):* High in protein, this yeasty, tofu-textured cake has a nutty flavor popular in Asian cooking. It slices like beef or chicken, so it's great for stir-frying. Tempeh is fully cooked, so just slice and heat. You can also marinate tempeh before heating, because it literally soaks up the flavors of the marinade.
- *Textured vegetable protein (TVP):* TVP is defatted soy protein that is in flake form. TVP makes a great substitute for ground beef in soups, stews, spaghetti, sloppy joes, and chili.
- *Tofu:* Also called soybean curd or bean curd, tofu is made from curdled soymilk, which is taken from ground, cooked soybeans. Tofu is white, and the texture varies from that of custard—smooth and creamy—

to much firmer versions. It is bland, which gives tofu the ability to taste like the food with which it is being cooked. Like tempeh, its blandness makes it great for marinating. Try to use light tofu, which saves calories and fat grams for sauces that can add flavor to your meal.

The Great Grains

You hear so much about using whole-grain instead of white bread. Not only do grains give your meal more texture and flavor, but they are rich in the notable nutrients folic acid, vitamin B_6, iron, and zinc. Here, we give you a crash course in whole grains and help you learn how to use them.

- *Barley:* Loaded with the phytochemicals tocotrienol and lignan, barley comes in three different forms: pearled barley, which is the type most commonly eaten because it cooks much more quickly than the others but has actually been milled at least six times, removing all the nutritious bran layers; scotch barley, or pot barley, has been milled about three times, making it more nutritious than pearled barley; hulled barley, the most nutritiously valuable of the three, is barley in its whole-grain form.
- *Bulgur (also bulgur wheat, bulghur):* As a form of whole wheat, bulgur retains the flavor of whole wheat as well. This Mediterranean staple has a chewy, tender texture.
- *Couscous:* This versatile food is made from granular semolina, a coarsely ground grain. It can be served with milk as porridge, with salad dressing as a salad mixed with vegetables as a main dish, or sweetened and mixed with fruits for dessert.
- *Millet:* This bland grain tends to pick up the flavor of the foods it is cooked with, yet it lends a crunch, giving an interesting texture to many dishes. Although it is used in the United States almost exclusively as animal and bird feed, a large portion of the world's population eats this wholesome grain.
- *Quinoa:* This tiny, bead-shaped seed is so incredibly rich in the health-promoting phytochemical saponin that it has a strong taste. It is similar to couscous, with an ivory color and a bland, delicate taste. It cooks similar to rice, expanding to four times its original size. Not actually a grain, quinoa (pronounced *KEEN-wa*) is low in gluten, which is good for those who need a gluten-free diet. Most

packaging suggests rinsing away the saponins before cooking, but we recommend not doing so to reap the possible heart disease prevention and cancer-fighting value of the phytochemical.

- *Rice:* Rice is classified by the size of the kernel: long-, medium-, and short-grained rice. Never rinse rice before cooking, as it washes away many of the nutrients. Stay away from rice packaged with sauces and spices because they tend to be higher in fat and salt. The following are some different varieties you'll find in your neighborhood market:
  - *White rice:* The most stripped down version of the grain—the husk, germ, and bran layers have been milled. It is the form most Americans eat. It is of much less nutritional value than the whole grain.
  - *Wild rice:* Not really rice at all, it is a marsh grass. It is important to clean wild rice well before preparing it. Wild rice has a chewy texture and nutty taste.
  - *Brown rice:* Mild and pleasant-tasting, this is the form that has the greatest amount of fiber and nutrients, although the hull and part of the bran have been removed. It's light tan in color with a chewy texture and nutlike flavor. Allow extra cooking time when using brown rice.

Grain Gallery

Grain	Calories per 1 Cup Cooked	Protein per 1 Cup Cooked	Fat per 1 Cup Cooked	Fiber per 1 Cup Cooked	Rich in These Nutrients
Barley	270	7.42 g	2.16 g	13.6 g	Thiamin, niacin, vitamin B_6, vitamin E, copper, iron, magnesium, manganese, phosphorus, zinc, selenium
Bulgur	151.06	5.61 g	0.44 g	8.19 g	Niacin, vitamin B_6, folic acid, pantothenic acid, magnesium, manganese, zinc
Millet	285.6	8.42 g	2.40 g	3.12 g	Thiamin, riboflavin, niacin, vitamin B_6, folic acid, iron, magnesium, manganese, phosphorus, zinc
Couscous	175.84	5.95 g	0.25 g	2.20 g	Niacin, thiamin, selenium

Grain	Calories per 1 Cup Cooked	Protein per 1 Cup Cooked	Fat per 1 Cup Cooked	Fiber per 1 Cup Cooked	Rich in These Nutrients
Quinoa	317.90	11.14 g	4.93 g	5.02 g	Thiamin, riboflavin, niacin, vitamin E, copper, iron, manganese, magnesium, zinc, potassium
White rice	161.7	3.42 g	0.26 g	0.99 g	Thiamin, riboflavin, niacin
Wild rice	165.64	6.54 g	0.56 g	2.95 g	Thiamin, riboflavin, niacin, vitamin B_6, folic acid, copper, magnesium, manganese, phosphorus, zinc
Brown rice	216.45	5.05 g	1.75 g	3.51 g	Thiamin, niacin, vitamin B_6, iron, magnesium, manganese, phosphorus, selenium, zinc

g = gram(s).

The Beans

In keeping with life course dietary goals of reducing the amount of meat and poultry in your diet, we have endeavored to include many types of beans or legumes in our meals in the hopes that you'll give them a try. They are high in protein (one of the notable nutrients) and carry the side benefits that they are low in fat, have no saturated fat, and are a valuable source of fiber. And as a special benefit to pregnant women, many of them are rich in the other notable nutrients—folic acid, vitamin B_6, calcium, iron, and zinc. Here's the skinny on beans and their nutritional goodness:

- *Black beans:* Also called turtle beans, these are slightly sweet in flavor. They have a black skin and are cream colored inside.
- *Black-eyed peas:* These small beans, also called cowpeas, are tan and have a small black eye-shaped spot at the inside curve.
- *Chickpeas:* Also called garbanzo beans, these beans are round with a mildly nutty flavor. They are firm in texture and can be used hot or cold.
- *Great Northern beans:* These delicately flavored white beans can be used in cream sauces, soups, and stews.
- *Kidney beans:* These firm, full-bodied beans are often used as a base for chili. They are red on the outside with a light-colored flesh.

Eating for Life

As I have stressed throughout this book, your baby's time in utero is just a snippet of her or his *total life course*—albeit a very critical one. The infant, toddler, preschool, grade school, and teen years— just for starters—will greatly influence the expression of how genetics and life in the womb influences the health risks for your child-to-be. That's why we'd like to teach you how to eat *for long life and optimal health.* So although we've focused on making these meal plans perfect for you during your days in waiting, they are also a fabulous teaching tool for how you and your family should eat *all the time* to prevent disease and feel energetic.

You'll be learning that your life course eating style, before, during, and after your pregnancy should include

- More vegetarian meals
- More fruits and vegetables
- More whole-grain foods, such as brown rice, barley, bulgur, quinoa, and millet, and fewer refined grains, such as white bread, white rice, and pasta
- More fish
- More nuts and seeds (for their protein, vitamins, and minerals)
- Fewer and smaller portions of red meat (beef, pork, and lamb)
- Less saturated and *trans*-fatty acids—replace then with mono-unsaturated and polyunsaturated fats whenever possible

During pregnancy, it is also important to eat protein at every meal. Chapter Eleven contains more detailed information on how to accomplish these goals for your whole family.

- *Lentils:* These are red or brown and can be served cold or hot in soups or salads. These tiny disc-shaped beans are a popular substitute for meat, particularly in countries such as India.
- *Pinto beans:* Usually eaten as refried beans or red Mexican beans, these beans are reddish, streaked with pink. Use canned refried beans with caution, as they may be high in fat. Always opt for the low-fat versions, or try making your own.

- *Soybeans:* There are over 1,000 varieties of these legumes that vary in size depending on the variety. They come in many different colors, including red, green, yellow, black, and brown. They can be cooked, sprouted, or made into soy by-products.

Bean Bonanza

Beans, 1 Cup Cooked	Calories	Protein	Fat	Fiber	Rich in These Nutrients
Black beans	227.04	15.24 g	0.93 g	14.96 g	Thiamin, folic acid, copper, iron, magnesium, manganese, phosphorus, potassium, zinc
Black-eyed peas	199.52	13.3 g	0.91 g	11.18 g	Thiamin, riboflavin, vitamin C, magnesium
Chickpeas	285.60	11.88 g	2.74 g	10.56 g	Vitamin B_6, vitamin C, folic acid, pantothenic acid, copper, iron, magnesium, manganese, phosphorus, potassium, selenium, sodium, zinc
Great Northern beans	208.86	14.74 g	0.80 g	12.39 g	Thiamin, vitamin B_6, folic acid, calcium, copper, iron, magnesium, manganese, phosphorus, potassium, selenium, zinc
Kidney beans	207.36	13.31 g	0.79 g	8.96 g	Thiamin, riboflavin, niacin, folic acid, copper, iron, magnesium, manganese, phosphorus, potassium, zinc
Lentils	229.68	17.86 g	0.75 g	15.64 g	Thiamin, riboflavin, niacin, vitamin B_6, folic acid, pantothenic acid, copper, iron, magnesium, manganese, phosphorus, potassium, selenium, zinc

(continued)

Bean Bonanza (*continued*)

Beans, 1 Cup Cooked	Calories	Protein	Fat	Fiber	Rich in These Nutrients
Pinto beans	206.40	11.66 g	1.94 g	11.04 g	Thiamin, riboflavin, vitamin B_6, vitamin E, folic acid, calcium, copper, iron, magnesium, manganese, phosphorus, potassium, selenium, sodium, zinc
Soybeans, green	253.80	22.32 g	11.52 g	7.56 g	Thiamin, riboflavin, niacin, vitamin C, folic acid, calcium, copper, iron, magnesium, manganese, phosphorus, potassium, zinc

g = gram(s).

FABULOUS FLAVORING SECRETS

Flavoring food naturally—with little added fat and being stingy with the salt shaker—can offer many health advantages. Even though it may be tough to part ways with butter, margarine, and salt as the main topping for vegetables, rice, potatoes, and other foods, you'll soon find much enjoyment in learning how to use other flavoring secrets. Here, we share one of Karin's and two of Kris's favorite flavoring secrets.

Karin's Provençal Herb Mix

Residing part of the time in Europe, I have become accustomed to simply tossing a bag of Herbes de Provençe in my grocery basket. I love using it on salads, vegetables, in soups—and just about anything edible! In the States, it is more difficult—though not impossible—to find the premixed variety. So Kris has taken the ingredients in Herbes de Provence and developed a recipe that you can use—see page 91. Keep the mix in a jar in your pantry—it will last for about 6 months. I recommend sprinkling some on salads, veggies, rice, grains, soups, and other bounties of nature.

Kris's Flavoring Secret #1: Cooking with Wine

At first glance, you may think that it's not such a great idea to even mention wine in a book that has to do with pregnancy. Indeed, women even thinking about getting pregnant should abstain from all alcohol.

Karin's Provençal Herb Mix

Mix equal parts of each herb in its dried state:

- *Basil:* Part of the mint family, basil may be used dried but is much more flavorful when fresh leaves are used. It is a staple of Mediterranean cooking, especially in Italian dishes.
- *Fennel seed:* Also called finocchio, fennel has stems that resemble a celery stalk and has a bulbous base. Both the stem and the base can be eaten. The seeds, greenish brown in color, are the part that is used in Herbes de Provence.
- *Lavender flowers:* The original recipe calls for lavender flowers. If you can find them, they will add a delicate, distinct flavor to this herbal blend.
- *Marjoram:* A popular member of the mint family variety is sweet marjoram, which is found in stores simply as marjoram. This herb has pale green, oval leaves and a sweet, mild flavor.
- *Rosemary:* This needle-shaped herb also belongs to the mint family. It's grayish green in color and has a lemony aroma mixed with a hint of pine. Use both fresh and dried.
- *Sage:* This herb has a bitter and musty mint taste. Its leaves are greenish gray. Sage also contains the phytochemical luteolin, a potential cancer fighter.
- *Savory:* Closely related to the mint family, savory has a flavor and smell between those of thyme and mint. There are two types, summer and winter; summer is slightly milder than winter.
- *Thyme:* Another mint relative, this herb has a minty yet light lemon-flavored taste. Thyme contains the phytochemical luteolin, which means it may help fight cancer.

However, using wine when cooking is a wonderful way to lend a rich flavor to food, without having any alcohol at all. That's right—when you add small amounts of wine to soups or stews (or anything hot), the alcohol evaporates off rather quickly, and you're left with the deep, rich flavor in which it was seated.

Kris's Flavoring Secret #2: Bouillons

No doubt you'll notice that Kris uses three different types of bouillon granules in her recipes: regular, 33% reduced sodium, and very low sodium. There is a method to this seeming madness! Vegetable, beef, and chicken bouillon granules are fabulous flavoring additives. The problem with the regular variety of bouillon granules is the sodium content: 1 teaspoon has 900 milligrams of sodium. To bump up the flavor, Kris often wants to use more than that amount in her recipes, which would, of course, make some dishes prohibitively high in sodium. Instead, she carefully selects a reduced-sodium version. This way, the flavor is awesomely high and the sodium is delicately balanced. You'll see the 33% reduced sodium variety (600 milligrams sodium per teaspoon of bouillon) and the very low sodium version, (5 milligrams sodium per teaspoon of bouillon). Don't worry about having them both on hand, as they keep for approximately 1 year when well sealed.

How to Use Our Meal Plans

You'll see that our meal plans are not the regular one-size-fits-all type. Not only does each of the three trimester meal plans have two different calorie levels, but the prepregnancy trimester plan has three levels. Read through the guidelines below and you'll see that following them is as easy as can be, and as delicious.

First, consult the "Calorie Madness" section of Chapter Three (pages 64–65) to find out what calorie level you need to follow. Next, turn to the meal plan for your stage of pregnancy and note the foods included for that day for your calorie level. You'll see that sometimes the foods or portions differ, depending on the calorie level, and sometimes they are the same. Also, you may be adding or subtracting calories from your meal plan if you are losing or gaining weight too quickly. Note that all meal plan items in italics signify recipes that you'll find in Chapter Ten, listed by recipe type—for example, "Soups and Salads" or "Desserts, Smoothies, Shakes, and Snacks."

If you come upon a meal that doesn't appeal to you—we understand that some people just don't like tuna fish sandwiches, for example—bear in mind that, as we said earlier, every breakfast, lunch, and dinner is equivalent caloriewise with every other breakfast, lunch, and dinner, within the same calorie level and the same trimester. So you could swap your sandwich with a lunch from another day, maybe with a Guacamole Wrap or a Peanut Papaya Pasta Salad. Or you could just follow another complete day of the meal plan. In the next section, you'll read about a third option: designing your own meal plans. For the often difficult first trimester, we've provided you with one additional option. At the end of our meal plans in this trimester you'll find several alternative meals designed especially for the needs of the mother suffering from morning sickness. Though these meals do not offer as much variety as is optimal, on bad days they may be all you can manage and are infinitely better than eating nothing.

The final section of each meal plan day gives you the nutritional rundown on what you've eaten. We've included information on calories, protein, carbohydrates, fiber, fat, percent of calories from fat, fat types (saturated, monounsaturated, and polyunsaturated), and amounts of the notable nutrients. Please be aware that each meal of each day is fabulously healthy, whether you are pregnant or not—you might even want to follow our prepregnancy trimester meal plans when you are no longer pregnant, to lose or gain weight or just to help you eat healthily.

How to Make Your Own Meal Plans

As I mentioned above, we have provided the tools you'll need to design your own meal plans, whether you want to do this every day or just occasionally. It can be useful for special occasions such as Thanksgiving, if you are growing vegetables that you want to incorporate into your diet, or even if you have caught a fish you want to eat!

Each trimester chapter contains a table that specifies how many servings of each food group are needed daily for each calorie level. First, find the calorie level you are following and then see what number of servings are allocated for each food group: nonfat dairy foods, whole-grain foods, legumes, fruits, vegetables, lean proteins, nuts or seeds, and added fats. Check the list of serving sizes on the next page to find out how much constitutes a serving for each food.

For your convenience, in each trimester chapter we also provide a table of our recommendations for how the foods can be allocated throughout the day. Of course, you don't need to follow these tables exactly, but they are specially designed to take into account your changing appetite in each trimester.

What Is in a Serving?

Fruits
- 1 medium-size piece of fruit
- ¾ cup berries
- 1 cup melon chunks
- ½ cup grapes
- ½ cup juice
- ¼ cup nectar

Vegetables
- 1 cup raw greens (spinach, romaine, and so on)
- ½ cup cooked greens
- 1 cup raw cut-up vegetables (such as broccoli)
- ½ cup cooked cut-up vegetables (such as broccoli)
- ¼ cup starch vegetables (corn, peas, lima beans)
- 1 carrot
- 2 stalks celery or bok choy

Legumes and Soy Products
- ½ cup cooked beans or lentils (such as black beans or pinto beans)
- 3 ounces tofu
- 3 ounces tempeh
- ¼ cup soy nuts

Starches and Breads
- ½ cup cooked rice, pasta, or other grain (such as quinoa)
- ½ cup cooked cereal (oatmeal, cream of wheat)
- 1 slice bread
- 1 whole English muffin
- ¾ cup dry cereal
- ½ large pita bread
- ⅓ bakery-size bagel
- 5 saltine crackers
- 2 crispbreads

Meat, Fish, Poultry, Low-Fat Cheese, and Eggs
- 1 ounce cooked low-fat beef, pork, poultry, or fish
- ¼ cup nonfat or reduced-fat cottage cheese (choose calcium fortified, if possible)

- 1 ounce reduced-fat cheese
- 1 ounce reduced-fat soy cheese
- 1 egg or 2 egg whites or ¼ cup liquid egg substitute

Milk, Yogurt, and Soymilk
- 1 cup skim milk
- 80 to 120 calorie yogurt (read labels)
- 1 cup reduced-fat soy milk (fortified with calcium and vitamins B_{12} and C)

Serving-Size Savvy

Note that one serving of a particular food group does not necessarily have the same amount of calories as one serving of another food. At first glance, in fact, you may think that Kris has planned too much food. But rest assured, she planned each day very carefully. The most each day's total will vary by is 3% of the target calorie level. Paying attention to serving sizes, though, is the only way you can make this work. Because this is so important, let's go over a few examples of how "just a little extra helping" can cause excessive weight gain; then we'll outline some tricks of the trade and give you some visual serving size help:

- The Best Hamburger makes a great dinner at 500 calories and 31 grams of fat. Use too much meat, though—just 1.5 ounces extra (4.5 ounces instead of 3 ounces per serving)—and you're eating 600 calories and 38 grams of fat. That's 100 extra calories and 7 extra grams of fat!
- Our delicious and nutritious Banana Split is a fabulous treat with 391 calories and 12 grams of fat. If you go overboard, though, and use an extra ½ cup ice cream, an extra tablespoon of almonds, and an extra tablespoon of chocolate syrup, you're eating 584 calories and 22 grams fat. That's 193 extra calories and 10 extra grams of fat!

I recommend that you measure very carefully for at least the first week you follow the Optimal Pregnancy Diet. Then you may find that you need to measure strictly only 1 day per week. Only you'll know for sure, however. An easy way to help you control your serving sizes is to measure the capacity of your favorite bowls, cups, and glasses. You may find that your favorite mug, filled 1 inch from the top, holds exactly 1 cup, perfect for measuring and drinking milk or juice. One last idea: Make it a habit to use measuring cups and measuring spoons to serve your food, rather than the conventional serving spoons that come with your cutlery. You'll find that serving yourself the appropriate amount becomes almost automatic.

The Scoop on Serving Sizes: A Visual Guide to Serving Sizes

Food	Number of Servings	Visual Size Equivalent
1 cup cooked rice or pasta	2 grain foods	Tennis ball
1 slice bread	1 grain food	CD case
1 cup raw fruit or vegetables	1 fruit or vegetable	Tennis ball
½ cup cooked fruit or vegetables	1 fruit or vegetable	Small fist
1 oz. cheese	1 high-fat protein	Pair of dice
1 tsp. olive oil	1 fat	Half-dollar
3 oz. cooked meat	3 protein	Deck of cards or cassette tape

oz. = ounce(s); tsp. = teaspoon(s).

HOW TO ENJOY THE 100-PLUS MOUTH-WATERING RECIPES IN THIS BOOK

What more could you ask for than 100-plus recipes created by culinary wizard Kris Napier and specially designed with the goals of the Optimal Pregnancy Diet in mind? You'll be surprised at their fabulous taste as well as their ability to help you harvest all the notable nutrients detailed in this book. Many of the dinner recipes serve two people, so that you can enjoy them with your partner or a friend. Most of the breakfasts and lunches serve just one, as we know you more commonly eat alone at these times. As for the shakes, smoothies, and other yummy snacks, the great majority also serve just one, but they can easily be doubled to share with a friend or loved one.

So that you can enjoy each recipe fully and not worry about overeating, we suggest you measure ingredients carefully, especially for such items as chocolate shakes, frozen lemonade, and banana splits. We have measured carefully and calculated the nutritional value of each recipe; you'll find the analysis at the end of each recipe. Note that the analysis includes any ingredients listed as optional.

The muffin recipes all yield 1 dozen to 2 dozen muffins. Don't worry about the excess; they freeze well.

What if I'm Not Gaining Weight?

In this section, Kris Napier has provided tables of healthy foods you can add if you are not gaining that optimal pound each week after the first trimester, or a pound every 2 to 4 weeks during the first trimester. Remember, don't try to add extra pounds with empty-calorie foods. Here, we've listed recommended weight-gain foods and serving sizes by food group. As we detailed in Chapter Three, add about 100 to 300 calories per day if you aren't gaining enough weight.

Nuts and Seeds

Food	Amount for About 100 Calories
Almonds	2 tsp. (0.6 oz. or 17 g)
Macadamia nuts	2 tsp. (0.5 oz. or 14 g)
Peanuts	2 tsp. (0.6 oz. or 17 g)
Pumpkin seeds	¼ cup + 2 tsp. (0.85 oz. or 24 g)
Soy nuts	¼ cup (0.75 oz. or 21 g)
Sunflower seeds	2 tsp. (0.6 oz. or 17 g)
Walnuts	2 tsp. (0.5 oz. or 14 g)

g = gram(s); oz. = ounce(s); tsp. = teaspoon(s).

Whole Grains

Food	Cooked Amount for About 100 Calories
Brown rice	½ cup
Bulgur	⅔ cup
Millet	⅓ cup
Quinoa	¼ cup cooked
Whole-grain bread	1½ slices
Whole-wheat bagel	¾ small bagel (1.5 oz. or 42 g)
Whole-wheat pita	½ pocket

g = gram(s); oz. = ounce(s).

Legumes

Food	Cooked Amount for About 100 Calories
Black beans	⅓ cup
Garbanzo beans	¼ cup + 2 tbsp.
Green soybeans	⅓ cup

(continued)

Legumes *(continued)*

Food	Cooked Amount for About 100 Calories
Kidney beans	⅓ cup
Lentils	⅓ cup
Soymilk	¾ cup

tbsp. = tablespoon(s).

Milk Products

Food	Amount for About 100 Calories
50% reduced-fat cheese	1.5 oz.
Low-fat cottage cheese	½ cup*
Skim milk	1¼ cups
Yogurt	½ cup*

*Because the calories in these foods can very greatly between brands,
  please read the labels to figure out how much to eat.

Lean Protein

Food	Cooked Amount for About 100 Calories
Egg whites	6
Egg, whole	1 has about 75 calories
Fish	3 oz.
Lean red meat*	2 oz.
Poultry*	2 oz.

*Please enjoy poultry no more than twice each week and lean meat no more
than twice each week.
oz. = ounce(s).

Fruits

Food	Amount for About 100 Calories
Apple	1¼ (6 oz. or 170 g)
Apricots	6 (7.5 oz. or 210 g)
Banana	1 (4 oz. or 113 g)
Berries	1⅔ cups
Cantaloupe	1⅔ cups
Grapes	1 cup
Orange	1½ (7 oz. or 198 g)
Papaya	1 (9 oz. or 250 g)
Pear	1 (6 oz. or 170 g)
Peach	2½ (8.5 oz. or 240 g)

g = gram(s); oz. = ounce(s).

WHAT IF I'M GAINING TOO MUCH WEIGHT?

If the scale indicates you are gaining weight too rapidly, then cut back your calories by about 100 per day, using the previous tables as a guide. You may need to cut down by 200 or even 300 calories to control your rate of weight gain. As I mentioned in Chapter Three, it is better to cut down on grain foods, fruit, and nuts and seeds, rather than protein and dairy foods. To avoid missing out on any vitamins and minerals, alternate the food group you cut down on and consider taking a vitamin and mineral supplement.

WHAT IF I'M VEGETARIAN OR VEGAN?

Our meal plans are especially easy to follow if you are vegetarian (eating no meat, poultry, fish, or other seafood) or vegan (eating no animal products, i.e. excluding also eggs and dairy products). As you'll notice, we emphasize the use of plant-based foods, which is the way health professionals recommend everyone should eat for optimal health and to prevent cancer, heart disease, and other chronic illnesses. When you do encounter meat, fish, poultry or dairy products, either consult the "Vegetarian and Vegan Substitution Chart" below for an equivalent food item to use instead or feel free to substitute a vegetarian lunch or dinner within the menu plan in that trimester. As mentioned earlier, all breakfasts, lunches, and dinners can be exchanged with each other within each trimester and calorie level. You may also wish to create your own menus as outlined in each trimester. Simply choose the vegan or vegetarian options from our lists of serving sizes for the different food groups starting on page 94 through 95.

Vegan and Vegetarian Substitution Chart

1 cup skim milk is equivalent to	⅔ cup low-fat fortified soymilk
1 oz. 50% reduced-fat cheese is equivalent to	1 oz. tofu cheese
1 cup yogurt is equivalent to	1½ cups low-fat fortified soymilk or 3 oz. tofu cheese
½ cup ice cream	½ cup tofutti frozen tofu dessert
3 oz. beef, pork, or chicken	1 cup low-fat tofu, ½ cup tempeh, ⅔ cup legumes
3 oz. fish	¾ cup low-fat tofu, ⅓ cup tempeh, ½ cup legumes

oz. = ounce(s).

Keep in mind that some of the notable nutrients, particularly iron and zinc, can be more difficult to obtain from a vegetarian or vegan diet, and you will need to plan your diet especially carefully to ensure an adequate protein and calcium intake if you are vegan. For this reason, foods with added vitamins or minerals, such as fortified breakfast cereal, soymilk, and calcium-enriched orange juice, can be very valuable. I would also encourage you to discuss with your health-care provider whether you should take a multivitamin and mineral supplement, particularly if you are vegan.

OTHER QUESTIONS

What if I'm Carrying Twins, Triplets, or . . . ?

You might not know you are carrying twins (or more) right away, especially if you did not take fertility drugs. If you start to gain weight quickly, especially if you are not eating excessively, you should ask your obstetrician or nurse midwife to check you for this possibility. Women who don't know they are carrying two or more babies might think they are gaining weight too quickly and thus might restrict food intake to slow the weight gain. This could result in undernourishing the babies.

Yes, you should gain more weight if you are carrying more than one baby. Mothers of twins should gain a total of 35 to 45 pounds, or about 1.5 pounds per week during the second and third trimesters; if you are carrying more than two babies, ask your doctor about weight gain. You'll need to gain more weight to support the babies' growth but also to support the extra growth required of the placenta or placentas. Also, because of the tremendous demand on your body to nourish two (or more) babies, you should take prenatal vitamins.

It is not uncommon for twins to be born early, at 37 to 38 weeks, instead of the normal 40 weeks' gestation. Your obstetrician will want to prevent early birth, though, by having you rest from a certain point of your pregnancy on; this is quite individual. Also, getting off your feet can improve blood flow to the babies and bring birth weight up to the healthy average.

Is There Any Healthy Fast Food for Those Hectic or Away-from-Home Moments?

We all have those times when we just cannot make it home to fix a meal. The problem with most fast food is that it is loaded with fat (especially saturated fat and *trans*-fatty acids) and sodium. There are some better choices, though. Most fast-food restaurants offer a grilled chicken sandwich. Just order it with extra tomatoes and extra lettuce (and onions if your stomach tolerates them); beware of added mayonnaise or fat-laden sauces. Add a side salad, requesting low-fat dressing, and skim milk. Another option is to hit the salad bar at the grocery store and load up a pile of lettuce with all the veggies you can; add some garbanzo beans for protein.

What Should I Drink?

We've included lots of milk and dairy products so that you get plenty of bone-building nutrients. We've also "used up" your calories in healthy foods you and your baby need. For extra beverages, we suggest you drink:

- Water—lots of it!
- Decaffeinated coffee or tea
- Calorie-free, artificial sweetener–free flavored fruit teas (raspberry tea, orange-ginger tea, etc.); do avoid herbal teas (see "Can I Use Herbal Products?" on the next page)
- Club soda or seltzer water that may be flavored but is calorie free

Why Do I Need Snacks?

You may read this more than once in this book, but it's so important we'd like to repeat it! The baby growing inside of you needs a continuous source of energy. That's why we'd like you to have three moderately sized meals and three snacks each day.

How Else Can I Optimize Calorie Intake?

Become an expert on healthy cooking strategies. Although this is always a great idea, cooking the lean, healthy, nutrient-loaded way is really key during pregnancy. Kris Napier is an expert at figuring out how to make any food gourmet style—but with considerably fewer calories and more nutrients than you'd expect. We'd like you to learn how to use fresh herbs, dried herbs, flavored vinegars, and broths in cooking, all of which are great flavor substitutes for the fat found in so many recipes.

How Much Should I Exercise?

Certainly, you want to adopt very healthy habits during pregnancy. This includes exercise: If you haven't been exercising, you may want to start now. But we don't want you to start anything that could injure you or your baby. If you want to begin exercising, remember *slow* and *gentle* and *gradual* as key words. A great way to exercise is to begin gentle strolling, working your way up to a walk and then a brisk walk. Always, though, check with your obstetrician or nurse midwife to make sure you are in shape for any change in your exercise habits. You might also check with your health-care provider about enrolling in a pregnancy exercise class that is led by an acknowledged expert in the field. If you have been exercising regularly, it is still a good idea to ask your physician or nurse midwife if you can continue in the same way.

Are Medications Safe?

We feel that this is such an important question that we would like you to discuss the use of any medication—prescription and over-the-counter (aspirin, Tylenol, cold and flu preparations, allergy medications, and so on)—with your obstetrician. Even if your general practitioner or family doctor prescribes a medication, check it out with your obstetrician.

Can I Use Herbal Products?

We suggest steering clear of herbal products during your pregnancy. Remember, they are touted for their physiological effects. Indeed, several do have powerful effects. The effects of most during pregnancy have not been studied, so we suggest avoiding all of them. If you do want to use an herbal product, be sure to consult your obstetrician first.

MOVING ONE STEP CLOSER TO IMPLEMENTING THE OPTIMAL PREGNANCY DIET

As you go forward to the chapter that meets your stage of pregnancy (or the months before), keep track of the important information that will help you translate our advice into food on your table. Mark sections that you find particularly helpful with sticky notes or dog-ear the pages—do whatever you need to make our Optimal Pregnancy Diet work for you.

CHAPTER FIVE

The Prepregnancy Optimal Diet

You may be surprised that there is such a thing as a prepregnancy diet. Traditionally, there hasn't been. But we believe that preparing your body for pregnancy and learning how to eat *before* you become pregnant is crucial, so we've added this preparatory trimester. Think of it as the in-training trimester—a time to learn about optimal eating before it becomes so essential.

There's another very important reason to train your body and your nutritional habits for pregnancy: to give yourself nutritional insurance. In the first days of pregnancy, you might not yet know you are pregnant. Even so, that microscopic baby inside of you will undergo amazingly complex construction projects—construction projects that demand the optimal amount of all nutrients. As you'll read in more detail in Chapter Six, at just 28 days after conception the baby's brain and spinal column are completely formed—and this requires that you get sufficient folic acid, protein, zinc, and vitamin B_6, four of the notable nutrients. As you can imagine, eating well before you become pregnant can help ensure that these nutrients are on board from the very moment you conceive.

We're still not done justifying the Prepregnancy Optimal Diet! We are a society very focused on appearances, a phenomenon that causes many women to skimp on eating and to therefore border on having nutrient deficiencies.

Surveys reveal that 75% of American women are dissatisfied with their appearance. Girls begin dieting as early as 9 or 10 years of age. By the time they are high school seniors, 90% of girls diet regularly, even though only between 10% and 15% are above the weight recommended by the standard height–weight charts. A U.S. Department of Agriculture survey revealed that 50% to 60% of American women get less than 70% of the recommended amounts of nutrients essential to pregnancy. Another recent survey found that only 30% of 250 women between the ages of 21 and 35 had normal bone mass. The researchers who conducted this study concluded that women are so afraid that eating dairy products will make them gain weight that they are starving themselves into osteoporosis.

So, as you can see, learning to eat well before pregnancy gives your body a chance to ensure sufficient levels of vitamins and minerals and even to build up some extra stores, which places you, your body, and your baby-to-be in a much better state for the nutrition marathon that pregnancy is.

NUTRITION PRIORITIES

The following are nutrition priorities during the prepregnancy phase:

- Achieving and maintaining an optimal body weight
- Learning to eat three meals and three snacks daily
- Increasing your intake of folic acid-rich foods
- Focusing on iron-rich foods
- Boosting your intake of calcium- and vitamin D–rich foods

Achieving and Maintaining an Optimal Body Weight

It is in these months before pregnancy that you should work on bringing your body weight closer to your recommended weight. Let's take a look at why this is so important.

If you are overweight (defined as having a body mass index [BMI] over 25; see Chapter Three), you should try to reduce your weight before you become pregnant. Once you are pregnant, you should still gain a minimum of 15 pounds even if you are very overweight. Gaining 25 pounds gives you a better chance of taking in all essential nutrients—and gives your baby the best chance of harvesting all the nutrients he or she needs to grow and develop optimally. There is another reason why it is important to drop excess weight before becoming pregnant: Women who begin pregnancy at a BMI greater than 29 have a much greater chance of pregnancy-related complications. These include pregnancy-induced hypertension (high blood pressure), pregnancy-induced preeclampsia (formerly known as toxemia), gestational diabetes, and delivery complications (including an increased likelihood of having to have a cesarean section delivery).

Being below your optimal weight (having a BMI less than 20; see Chapter Three) can lead to complications, too. Women who are underweight when they conceive are more likely to deliver an infant who has a birth weight below the expected average. As you read in Chapter One, babies with low birth weights may have higher risk of developing heart disease and diabetes as adults.

So use this training trimester to lose or gain weight to bring your BMI into or closer to the recommended range of 20 to 25. To help you lose or gain healthfully (or maintain your weight), we have provided this training trimester's diet in three calorie levels: 1,700, 1,900, and 2,100. If you decide to drop some excess weight, do not eat fewer than 1,700 calories daily. Dropping your calorie intake more than this can seriously deplete your body of important nutrients, which can place you at risk nutritionally if you do become pregnant shortly after losing the weight. Instead, increase your level of physical activity, which will help you to lose the excessive body fat while maintaining and building up muscle tissue. If you want to give yourself some extra time before becoming pregnant, then you can drop down to 1,500 calories for a time. Don't lose more than 2 pounds per week, as a faster loss is even more likely to deplete your body of nutrients and can also lead to muscle loss along with fat loss. After losing some weight, go back up to a minimum of 1,700 calories to recharge your body nutritionally. No matter what calorie intake you follow to lose weight, be sure and take a vitamin and mineral supplement that supplies 100% of the U.S. RDA (Recommended Dietary Allowance) for all recommended nutrients. And remember that not only does regular exercise help you lose weight but it also helps you to lose fat rather than muscle mass.

If you need to gain weight, then follow the 2,100-calorie plan. If you aren't gaining 1 or 2 pounds each week, then increase your daily calorie intake by 100-calorie increments until you are gaining weight (see the tables of 100-calorie foods on pages 97–98). Just as with losing weight, it is not good to gain weight too quickly. Rapid weight gain generally translates into gaining more fat mass than muscle mass, which is not desirable. Regular exercise will help you gain muscle rather than fat.

Learning to Eat Three Meals and Three Snacks a Day

Though it may sound like a lot of food, we want you to get used to eating six times daily before you become pregnant. Whether you are simply maintaining your weight during this training trimester or gaining or losing weight, we'd like you to divide up your food into three meals and three snacks. The reason is an important one. Once you become pregnant, the baby inside you is very fussy about the kind of calories, or energy, he or she needs.

Even if you take in the optimal number of calories during any one day, the baby may not get the optimal energy source if you eat only once or twice or even three times during the day. This optimal energy source is glucose, which enters the bloodstream after eating. Within a couple of hours after eating, blood glucose levels fall to a level where there is none extra left for baby to use (we all need glucose in our bloodstream at all times, simply for the body to function and the brain to work). When there is no extra glucose left, the baby's body then calls for more energy from the mom's stores. But there is a problem with using energy from the mom's fat stores: The cost of accessing this energy is the production of a by-product called ketones. Although ketones in normal amounts aren't a problem for the mom, they are not so great for the baby. This is why it is so important to eat frequently: Doing so keeps enough extra glucose in the bloodstream for baby to access at all times.

Training yourself to eat three meals and three snacks now is a great way to establish this good habit for when you do become pregnant.

Increasing Your Intake of Folic Acid-Rich Foods

Of all the notable nutrients, you'll find that we remind you the most about folic acid. This B vitamin, found in citrus fruits and juices, dark green leafy vegetables, strawberries, bananas, papayas, and legumes such as soy products and black beans, can reduce the incidence of spina bifida and other neural tube defects (defects of the spinal column). According to the U.S. Centers for Disease Control and Prevention (CDC), if all women capable of becoming pregnant consumed 400 micrograms of folic acid daily, 50% to 70% of all cases of spina bifida and anencephaly (a more serious type of neural tube defect) would be prevented.

The key is getting enough of this nutrient during the time that you are just *thinking* about becoming pregnant. As you read earlier in this chap-

ter, within just 4 weeks after you conceive, the baby's brain and spinal column are completely formed. As we've also said before, many women may
not even know they are pregnant when this critically important construction project is taking place. This is why, in fact, the CDC recommends
that all women take in at least 400 micrograms of folic acid—and possibly
as much as 600 micrograms—during their childbearing years.

Folic acid remains an essential nutrient throughout pregnancy, helping
baby complete all construction projects. Then, as the mom approaches
delivery, folic acid pops up again in importance for another reason: Folic
acid can help prevent premature delivery. So getting in the habit of eating
folic acid–rich foods is a great help to you throughout your pregnancy.

As you know by now, we are not concerned just about you and baby
during your pregnancy: We are also concerned about your (meaning yours
and baby's) life course, or everything that impacts your health throughout
life. Research suggests that getting enough folic acid can help reduce the
risk of some cancers, as well as heart disease.

Focusing on Iron-Rich Foods

Many women have a difficult time consuming 15 milligrams of iron daily,
the recommended intake for women during their menstruating years.
Imagine how difficult it is when iron requirements increase to 30 milligrams during pregnancy! This is one reason we want you to boost your
intake of iron-rich foods during this training trimester. But there's another
important reason.

If you are like many women in America, you may not be outright anemic,
but you may border on anemia. When you become pregnant, increased
iron needs can push you over the edge and make you anemic. For this
additional reason, we'd like you to boost iron intake now. Good sources
include whole-grain foods, legumes, and lean meat. Iron from nonmeat
sources will be better absorbed if you eat a vitamin C–rich food such as
citrus fruits, berries, or tomatoes at the same time.

Boosting Intake of Calcium- and Vitamin D–Rich Foods

As mentioned earlier, many women cut dairy foods from their eating
plans in an attempt to cut calories. According to the National Osteoporosis Foundation, the typical American diet provides less than 600 milligrams of calcium per day, a little over half the recommended amount. As

a result, an alarming two thirds of women have less than optimal bone mass. Before we detail how much calcium you should be getting, let's review a few bone basics.

The skeleton is much like the steel framework of a skyscraper: It supports body tissues just as steel upholds the building. But the skeletal bones are distinctly different from lifeless metal. Like other tissues, bones are very much alive and constantly changing in a process called remodeling. Just as skin constantly sloughs off old cells and lays down new cells, old bone is constantly broken down and new bone is built up.

Two types of cells are critical to this process. *Osteoclasts* break down and carry away old bone, whereas *osteoblasts* bring in new bone cells. Surprisingly, bones grow well into the third decade of life, simply because the balance remains in favor of the osteoblasts until this time. Although they stop growing in length during adolescence, bones bulk up, or increase in density, until somewhere between age 25 and 35. Getting enough calcium throughout this entire bone-building process is critically important. Calcium intake, in fact, is one of the most important predictors of bone strength. That's why calcium requirements increase as children grow in size but then stay high throughout the autumn stages of life.

Recently, the Food and Medicine Board of the Institute of Medicine of the National Academy of Sciences, the health authority that sets nutrition requirements, reset calcium requirements, making them higher for the entire population. This was based on new research revealing that calcium requirements are greater than previously thought. The new requirements are called Dietary Reference Intakes (DRIs) instead of RDAs. The requirements are as follows:

- Infants 0 to 6 months, 210 milligrams
- Infants 6 to 12 months, 270 milligrams
- Children 1 to 3 years, 500 milligrams
- Children 4 to 8 years, 800 milligrams
- Children 9 to 18 years, 1,300 milligrams
- Men and women, 19 to 50 years, 1,000 milligrams
- Men and women, 51-plus years, 1,200 milligrams
- Pregnant and lactating women, 14 to 18 years, 1,300 milligrams
- Pregnant and lactating women, 19-plus, 1,000 milligrams

Calcium is important to males and females of all ages, but it is especially critical to women, the population most severely afflicted by osteoporosis.

Eighty percent of osteoporosis victims are female, for two main reasons. The first is just a matter of biology. Before menopause, women produce estrogen, a hormone that is important for a number of reasons. Among these reasons: Estrogen helps a woman hold on to bone mass. After menopause, when estrogen production stops, women can lose 2% to 5% of their bone mass each year. The second reason has to do with pregnancy: If a woman does not take in enough calcium during pregnancy, the developing baby will pull calcium out of the mom's bones, which decreases bone mass even further.

So to avoid being one of the 28 million American women affected by osteoporosis, start getting enough calcium today. Try eating calcium-rich dairy foods such as milk and yogurt. Even if you had no plans of becoming pregnant, this is an action that would favorably affect your life course.

THE PREPREGNANCY OPTIMAL DIET

Starting with these months before pregnancy, we've made getting all the nutrients you need much simpler, even in these days when you are just planning to become pregnant. In the pages that follow, we provide 2 weeks' worth of meal plans at three different calorie levels: 1,700, 1,900 and 2,100 calories. You just need to decide on the calorie level that best meets your needs now and then follow that plan. Unless you need to gain or lose weight, 1,900 is probably right for you. Fine-tune by adding or subtracting 100-calorie foods as outlined in the tables on pages 97 through 98.

The beauty of these meal plans is that every breakfast is exchangeable with every other breakfast, every lunch with every other lunch, and every dinner with every other dinner. With 14 different options for each meal, you can form myriads of meal plans for each day of this training trimester. (This is true for each of the trimesters of pregnancy.) Here, each breakfast has 400 calories, each lunch has 500 calories, and each dinner has 550 calories. Note that all meal plan items in italics signify recipes that you'll find in Chapter Ten. Enjoy!

Day 1		
	1,700 Calories	**1,900 Calories**	**2,100 Calories**

	1,700 Calories	**1,900 Calories**	**2,100 Calories**
Breakfast	*Cheesy Mushroom Omelet*		
	2 slices whole-wheat toast with 1 tsp. margarine		
	1 cup skim milk		
Morning Snack	1 papaya (approximately 11 oz. or 300 g)		
Lunch	*Salad of Many Greens (Meal)*		
	½ cup calcium-fortified orange juice		
Afternoon Snack	¼ cup roasted pumpkin seeds	½ cup roasted pumpkin seeds	½ cup roasted pumpkin seeds, 1½ cups skim milk
Dinner	1 serving of *Ten-Minute Chicken Stir-Fry*		
	½ cup long-grain brown rice		
Evening Snack	1 cup skim milk	1½ cups skim milk, 1 favorite flavor Newton cookie	*Chocolate Shake*

Daily Nutrition Totals			
Calories	1,773	1,939	2,117
Protein (g)	105	112	120
Carbohydrates (g)	226	249	291
Fiber (g)	41	42	43
Fat (g)	52	57	55
% calories from fat	26	26	23
Distribution of fat type:			
Saturated	14%	18%	16%
Monounsaturated	57%	55%	58%
Polyunsaturated	29%	27%	26%
Vitamin B_6 (mg)	1.82	1.86	1.86
Folic acid (mcg)	521	527	527
Calcium (mg)	1,235	1,361	1,611
Iron (mg)	16	17	17
Zinc (mg)	9	11	11

g = gram(s); mcg = microgram(s); mg = milligram(s); oz. = ounce(s); tsp. = teaspoon.

Day 2		
1,700 Calories	*1,900 Calories*	*2,100 Calories*

Breakfast	1 small whole-wheat bagel with 2 tbsp. low-fat cream cheese		
	1 cup calcium-fortified orange juice		
Morning Snack	1 fresh orange	*Trail Mix I*	1½ cups calcium-fortified orange juice
Lunch	*Rice and Asparagus Salad*		
	Decaf fruit-flavored iced tea		
Afternoon Snack	Seltzer water with lemon or lime		*Trail Mix I*
Dinner	1 serving of *Ginger-Seared Chilean Sea Bass*		
	1 serving of *Celery and Apple Salad*		
	1 cup skim milk		
Evening Snack	1 cup Multi-Grain Cheerios with 1 cup skim milk	1½ cups Multi-Grain Cheerios with 1 cup skim milk	1½ cups Multi-Grain Cheerios with 1½ cups skim milk

Daily Nutrition Totals			
Calories	1,718	1,921	2,124
Protein (g)	83	88	91
Carbohydrates (g)	286	321	364
Fiber (g)	35	36	36
Fat (g)	35	41	41
% calories from fat	17	18	17
Distribution of fat type:			
Saturated	26%	29%	29%
Monounsaturated	42%	40%	40%
Polyunsaturated	32%	31%	31%
Vitamin B_6 (mg)	2.99	3.25	3.48
Folic acid (mcg)	664	700	768
Calcium (mg)	1,430	1,434	1,976
Iron (mg)	23	28	29
Zinc (mg)	13	16	16

g = gram(s); mcg = microgram(s); mg = milligram(s); tbsp. = tablespoon(s).

Day 3			
	1,700 Calories	**1,900 Calories**	**2,100 Calories**
Breakfast	1 serving of *Nutty Kiwi Salad*		
	2 slices whole-wheat toast with 2 tsp. margarine		
Morning Snack	1½ cups calcium-fortified orange juice		¼ cup roasted sunflower seeds, 3 fresh apricots (or 6 halves canned in juice)
Lunch	1 *Tofu Egg Salad Sandwich*		
	½ cup skim milk		
	1 fresh peach		
	1 serving of *Chocolate Fudge Brownies*		
Afternoon Snack	3 fresh apricots (or 6 halves canned in juice)		3 favorite flavor Newton cookies, 1½ cups skim milk
Dinner	1 serving of *Crock-Pot Flank Steak and Mushrooms*		
	½ cup skim milk		
Evening Snack	1 favorite flavor Newton cookie, decaf tea or coffee	2 favorite flavor Newton cookies, 1 cup skim milk	*Orange Shake*

Daily Nutrition Totals			
Calories	1,756	1,901	2,228
Protein (g)	80	90	111
Carbohydrates (g)	255	277	303
Fiber (g)	32	33	37
Fat (g)	51	52	70
% calories from fat	25	24	28
Distribution of fat type:			
Saturated	36%	37%	30%
Monounsaturated	40%	40%	34%
Polyunsaturated	24%	23%	36%
Vitamin B$_6$ (mg)	1.67	1.77	2.04
Folic acid (mcg)	436	448	508

Calcium (mg)	1,189	1,490	1,732
Iron (mg)	17	18	19
Zinc (mg)	13	14	17

g = gram(s); mcg = microgram(s); mg = milligram(s); tsp. = teaspon(s).

Day 4			
	1,700 Calories	*1,900 Calories*	*2,100 Calories*
Breakfast	1 poached egg		
	2 slices whole-wheat toast with 1 tsp. margarine		
	1 cup fresh raspberries		
	1 cup skim milk		
Morning Snack	1 banana	1 banana with 2 tsp. natural peanut butter	1 banana with 2 tsp. natural peanut butter and ¼ cup raisins
Lunch	1 serving of *Simple Garden Salad*		
	Five-Minute Tortilla		
	1 cup skim milk		
	1 fresh apricot (or 2 halves canned in juice)		
Afternoon Snack	Hot decaf tea, plain or flavored	¼ cup roasted sunflower seeds	⅓ cup roasted sunflower seeds
Dinner	1 serving of *Roasted Chicken and Veggies*		
	½ cup skim milk		
Evening Snack	¼ cup roasted sunflower seeds	Tea or Café Latte: 1 cup decaffeinated plain or flavored tea or flavored coffee with 1 cup skim milk	

Daily Nutrition Totals			
Calories	1,728	1,876	2,062
Protein (g)	107	118	122
Carbohydrates (g)	244	258	293

Daily Nutrition Totals (*continued*)			
Fiber (g)	48	49	52
Fat (g)	43	49	55
% calories from fat	22	23	23
Distribution of fat type:			
Saturated	21%	20%	19%
Monounsaturated	33%	36%	34%
Polyunsaturated	46%	44%	47%
Vitamin B$_6$ (mg)	3.07	3.21	3.39
Folic acid (mcg)	538	566	593
Calcium (mg)	1,191	1,498	1,526
Iron (mg)	17	18	19
Zinc (mg)	11	12	13

g = gram(s); mcg = microgram(s); mg = milligram(s); tsp. = teaspoon(s).

Day 5

	1,700 Calories	1,900 Calories	2,100 Calories
Breakfast	½ cup Fiber One cereal with 1 cup skim milk, 1 sliced banana, and ¼ cup raisins		
Morning Snack	1 serving of *Ready-to-go Fruit Salad*		
Lunch	Turkey Sandwich: 3 oz. lean turkey, 1 large romaine lettuce leaf, 2 tomato slices, and 1 tsp. mustard on 2 slices whole-wheat bread		
	1 cup skim milk		
	1 tangerine		
	1 shortbread cookie		
Afternoon Snack	Tall glass of herbal iced tea		2 oz. oat bran pretzels, tall glass of iced water with lemon or lime slice
Dinner	1 serving of *Vegetarian Chili*		
	1 serving of *Corny Cornbread*		
	½ cup skim milk		

	1,700 Calories	1,900 Calories	2,100 Calories
Evening Snack	Tea Latté: 1 cup decaffeinated plain or flavored tea with 1½ cups skim milk	1 *Banana Chocolate Chip Muffin*, 1 cup skim milk	

Daily Nutrition Totals			
Calories	1,715	1,926	2,152
Protein (g)	92	94	99
Carbohydrates (g)	289	324	368
Fiber (g)	48	52	56
Fat (g)	32	40	44
% calories from fat	16	18	17
Distribution of fat type:			
Saturated	25%	26%	26%
Monounsaturated	56%	57%	57%
Polyunsaturated	19%	17%	17%
Vitamin B$_6$ (mg)	3.28	3.39	3.39
Folic acid (mcg)	433	451	451
Calcium (mg)	1,544	1,433	1,433
Iron (mg)	17	19	20
Zinc (mg)	11	11	11

g = gram(s); mcg = microgram(s); mg = milligrams; oz. = ounce(s); tsp = teaspoon(s)

Day 6			
	1,700 Calories	**1,900 Calories**	**2,100 Calories**
Breakfast	2 *Cranberry Pumpkin Muffins* 1 cup favorite decaf plain or flavored tea		
Morning Snack	Hot flavored coffee	¼ cup soy nuts	½ cup soy nuts, 1½ cups calcium-fortified orange juice
Lunch	Roast Beef Sandwich: 4 oz. lean roast beef, 1 large romaine leaf, 2 tomato slices, and 2 tsp. light mayonnaise on 2 slices whole-wheat bread		

Day 6 (continued)

	1,700 Calories	1,900 Calories	2,100 Calories
Lunch (cont.)	1 serving of Cucumber Salad		
	1 cup skim milk		
Afternoon Snack	¼ cup soy nuts	Iced Café Latte: 1 cup skim milk with 1 cup iced flavored coffee	
Dinner	3 oz. grilled salmon		
	1 small baked potato with 2 tbsp. fat-free sour cream and 2 tbsp. chives		
	6 asparagus spears with 1 tsp. lemon juice		
	1 cup skim milk		
	1 kiwi		
Evening Snack	Café Latte: 1 cup skim milk with 1 cup decaf flavored coffee	¼ cup dry roasted peanuts	

Daily Nutrition Totals			
Calories	1,658	1,872	2,137
Protein (g)	118	127	135
Carbohydrates (g)	224	232	276
Fiber (g)	16	19	20
Fat (g)	35	53	58
% calories from fat	19	25	24
Distribution of fat type:			
Saturated	29%	23%	22%
Monounsaturated	45%	48%	46%
Polyunsaturated	26%	29%	32%
Vitamin B$_6$ (mg)	2.41	2.51	2.75
Folic acid (mcg)	403	456	568
Calcium (mg)	1,501	1,521	1,975
Iron (mg)	12	13	15
Zinc (mg)	14	15	16

g = gram(s); mcg = microgram(s); mg = milligram(s); oz. = ounce(s); tbsp. = tablespoon(s); tsp. = teaspoon(s).

Day 7

	1,700 Calories	1,900 Calories	2,100 Calories
Breakfast	1½ cups Raisin Bran cereal with 1 cup skim milk		
	1 pink grapefruit		
Morning Snack	Hot flavored coffee		¼ cup roasted pumpkin seeds with ¼ cup dried cranberries (Craisins)
Lunch	Chicken Pita: 3 oz. skinless chicken breast, ½ cup green peas, 2 tbsp. cilantro, and 2 tbsp. light mayonnaise in 1 whole-wheat pita pocket		
	½ cup grapes		
Afternoon Snack	Iced tea	1 cup fat-free vanilla yogurt with 1 cup sliced strawberries and 2 tbsp. wheat germ	1 cup fat-free vanilla yogurt with 1 cup sliced strawberries and 3 tbsp. wheat germ
Dinner	1 serving of *Cheesy Spinach Pizza*		
	½ cup calcium-fortified orange juice		
Evening Snack	*Creamy Orange Shake*		

Daily Nutrition Totals

Calories	1,698	1,891	2,080
Protein (g)	98	111	116
Carbohydrates (g)	265	298	331
Fiber (g)	27	33	36
Fat (g)	32	34	38
% calories from fat	16	16	16
Distribution of fat type:			
Saturated	20%	20%	20%
Monounsaturated	48%	46%	44%
Polyunsaturated	32%	34%	36%
Vitamin B$_6$ (mg)	2.87	3.11	3.18
Folic acid (mcg)	388	468	494
Calcium (mg)	1,259	1,538	1,553

Daily Nutrition Totals (continued)			
Iron (mg)	9	11	12
Zinc (mg)	8	11	14

g = gram(s); mcg = microgram(s); mg = milligram(s); oz. = ounce(s); tbsp. = tablespoon(s).

Day 8

	1,700 Calories	*1,900 Calories*	*2,100 Calories*
Breakfast	*Karin's Banana Breakfast Frappé* 2 slices whole-wheat toast with 2 tsp. favorite jam		
Morning Snack	Tall glass of ice water with lemon or lime	2 cups fresh or frozen raspberries	
Lunch	Peanut Butter Sandwich: 2 tbsp. natural peanut butter and 1 tbsp. favorite jam on 2 slices whole-wheat bread		
	1 cup skim milk		
	1 orange		
Afternoon Snack	1 serving of *Orange–Spinach Salad*		
Dinner	1 serving of *Sweet Potatoes in an Orange–Brown Sugar Glaze*		
	6 oz. grilled snapper		
	1 cup steamed green beans		
Evening Snack	Hot decaf plain or flavored tea	Tea Latté: 1 cup decaf plain or flavored tea with 1 cup skim milk	*Trail Mix I*, 1 cup skim milk

Daily Nutrition Totals			
Calories	1,751	1,957	2,165
Protein (g)	97	108	113
Carbohydrates (g)	249	290	328
Fiber (g)	34	51	54
Fat (g)	49	50	56
% calories from fat	24	22	22

Distribution of fat type:

Saturated	17%	17%	20%
Monounsaturated	47%	46%	45%
Polyunsaturated	36%	37%	35%
Vitamin B₆ (mg)	3.25	3.49	3.57
Folic acid (mcg)	758	835	860
Calcium (mg)	1,186	1,542	1,570
Iron (mg)	15	17	18
Zinc (mg)	9	11	12

g = gram(s); mcg = microgram(s); mg = milligram(s); oz. = ounce(s);
tbsp. = tablespoon(s); tsp. = teaspoon(s).

Day 9

	1,700 Calories	1,900 Calories	2,100 Calories
Breakfast	1 *Individual Pumpkin Pie Custard* with 3 tbsp. chopped walnuts		
	Tea Latté: 1 cup favorite decaf plain or flavored tea, 1 cup skim milk		
Morning Snack	1½ cups calcium-fortified orange juice		1 *Banana Chocolate Chip Muffin*
Lunch	1 serving of *Arugula with Basil–Balsamic Dressing*		
	1 cup skim milk		
	1 apple		
Afternoon Snack	Seltzer water with lemon or lime	1 *Banana Chocolate Chip Muffin*	2 cups low-fat microwave popcorn with 2 tbsp. fat-free parmesan cheese, 1½ cups calcium-fortified orange juice
Dinner	1 serving of *Ham and Mushroom Quiche*		
	1 serving of *Rainbow Side Salad*		
	½ cup skim milk		
Evening Snack	2 cups low-fat microwave popcorn with 2 tbsp. fat-free parmesan cheese		¼ cup walnuts

Daily Nutrition Totals			
Calories	1,697	1,946	2,136
Protein (g)	85	89	97
Carbohydrates (g)	258	298	302
Fiber (g)	40	44	45
Fat (g)	40	49	67
% calories from fat	21	22	27
Distribution of fat type:			
Saturated	20%	21%	17%
Monounsaturated	37%	41%	36%
Polyunsaturated	43%	38%	47%
Vitamin B$_6$ (mg)	2.02	2.17	2.34
Folic acid (mcg)	431	455	476
Calcium (mg)	1,346	1,376	1,394
Iron (mg)	14	16	17
Zinc (mg)	7	8	9

g = gram(s); mcg = microgram(s); mg = milligram(s); oz. = ounce(s); tbsp. = tablespoon(s).

Day 10			
	1,700 Calories	**1,900 Calories**	**2,100 Calories**
Breakfast		*Karin's Müsli*	
Morning Snack	Hot flavored coffee		*Karin's Banana Breakfast Frappé*, 2 tbsp. roasted sunflower seeds
Lunch		*Veggie Pita*	
		1 cup skim milk	
Afternoon Snack	Ice water with lemon or lime		1 serving of *Rainbow Side Salad*
Dinner		1 serving of *Salmon in a Tarragon–Orange Cream Sauce*	
		1 baked potato with 2 tbsp. low-fat sour cream	
		1 cup steamed broccoli with 1 tsp. margarine	
Evening Snack	*Karin's Banana Breakfast Frappé*		1 serving of *Chocolate Fudge Brownies*

Daily Nutrition Totals			
Calories	1,706	1,889	2,147
Protein (g)	88	92	98
Carbohydrates (g)	262	289	317
Fiber (g)	41	49	52
Fat (g)	40	49	63
% calories from fat	20	22	25
Distribution of fat type:			
Saturated	21%	20%	20%
Monounsaturated	36%	43%	40%
Polyunsaturated	43%	37%	40%
Vitamin B$_6$ (mg)	2.6	3	3.13
Folic acid (mcg)	401	525	573
Calcium (mg)	1,119	1,217	1,242
Iron (mg)	14	17	18
Zinc (mg)	8	9	10

g = gram(s); mcg = microgram(s); mg = milligram(s); tbsp. = tablespoon(s);
tsp. = teaspoon(s).

Day 11			
	1,700 Calories	*1,900 Calories*	*2,100 Calories*
Breakfast	1 whole-wheat English muffin with 2 tbsp. natural peanut butter		
	1 cup skim milk		
Morning Snack	Hot decaf plain or flavored tea	2 cups sliced strawberries	*Banana Smoothie*
Lunch	*Black Bean Avocado Wrap*		
	1 serving of *Chocolate Fudge Brownies*		
	½ cup skim milk		
Afternoon Snack	Seltzer water with lemon or lime	1 slice whole-wheat bread with 1 tsp. natural peanut butter	
Dinner	1 serving of *Roasted Red Pepper and Beef Wraps*		

Day 11 (continued)

	1,700 Calories	1,900 Calories	2,100 Calories
Dinner (cont.)		1 cup skim milk	
		2 apricots (or 4 halves canned in juice) and ½ cup blueberries with 2 tbsp. light whipped topping	
Evening Snack		Banana Smoothie	½ cup vanilla ice cream with 2 cups sliced strawberries

Daily Nutrition Totals			
Calories	1,764	1,963	2,096
Protein (g)	99	105	107
Carbohydrates (g)	271	308	324
Fiber (g)	36	46	46
Fat (g)	50	55	62
% calories from fat	23	23	24
Distribution of fat type:			
Saturated	28%	27%	32%
Monounsaturated	50%	49%	47%
Polyunsaturated	22%	24%	21%
Vitamin B$_6$ (mg)	2.11	2.37	2.4
Folic acid (mcg)	313	393	396
Calcium (mg)	1,543	1,613	1,697
Iron (mg)	15	17	17
Zinc (mg)	13	15	15

g = gram(s); mcg = microgram(s); mg = milligram(s); tbsp. = tablespoon(s); tsp. = teaspoon(s).

Day 12

	1,700 Calories	1,900 Calories	2,100 Calories
Breakfast		2 eggs, scrambled	
		1 slice whole-wheat toast with 2 tsp. margarine	
		1 cup skim milk	
Morning Snack		1 pink grapefruit	
Lunch		Carrot–Tuna Pita	
		1 cup calcium-fortified orange juice	

	1,700 Calories	1,900 Calories	2,100 Calories
Afternoon Snack	1 serving of *Rainbow Side Salad*		1 serving of *Rainbow Side Salad* sprinkled with ¼ cup roasted sunflower seeds
Dinner	1 serving of *Cream of Broccoli Soup*		
	1 serving of *Watercress–Date Salad*		
Evening Snack	Hot decaf flavored coffee	8 fresh dates	*Strawberry Milkshake*

Daily Nutrition Totals			
Calories	1,758	1,941	2,203
Protein (g)	83	85	103
Carbohydrates (g)	225	274	284
Fiber (g)	30	35	41
Fat (g)	63	63	81
% calories from fat	32	29	32
Distribution of fat type:			
Saturated	30%	31%	36%
Monounsaturated	46%	46%	40%
Polyunsaturated	23%	23%	34%
Vitamin B$_6$ (mg)	2.1	2.23	2.68
Folic acid (mcg)	568	577	720
Calcium (mg)	1,423	1,444	1,898
Iron (mg)	14	15	17
Zinc (mg)	8	8	12

g = gram(s); mcg = microgram(s); mg = milligram(s); tsp. = teaspoon(s).

Day 13

	1,700 Calories	1,900 Calories	2,100 Calories
Breakfast	*Peach Shake*		
	Small whole-wheat bagel with 1 tsp. natural peanut butter		
Morning Snack	Hot decaf plain or flavored tea		1 serving of *Ready-to-go Fruit Salad*

Day 13 (continued)

	1,700 Calories	1,900 Calories	2,100 Calories
Lunch	Garden Burger Supreme: one 3-oz. Garden Burger patty, 2 large romaine lettuce leaves, 4 cucumber slices, 1 tomato slice, and 1 tbsp. low-fat salad dressing on hamburger bun		
	1 cup skim milk		
	4 Hershey's Kisses		
Afternoon Snack	Ice water with lemon or lime	1 serving of *Refrigerator Fruit Salad*	1 serving of *Orange–Spinach Salad*
Dinner	1 serving of *Tuna Melt*		
	8 steamed asparagus spears		
	1 cup fresh or frozen raspberries with 1 tbsp. almonds		
Evening Snack	*Frozen Chocolate Banana Shake*		

Daily Nutrition Totals

Calories	1,726	1,876	2,112
Protein (g)	88	89	98
Carbohydrates (g)	300	338	355
Fiber (g)	46	50	58
Fat (g)	27	28	46
% calories from fat	14	13	18
Distribution of fat type:			
Saturated	34%	34%	25%
Monounsaturated	38%	37%	41%
Polyunsaturated	28%	29%	34%
Vitamin B$_6$ (mg)	2.15	2.47	3.03
Folic acid (mcg)	588	611	1,076
Calcium (mg)	1,300	1,343	1,590
Iron (mg)	14	15	21
Zinc (mg)	8	8	9

g = gram(s); mcg = microgram(s); mg = milligram(s); oz. = ounce(s);
tbsp. = tablespoon(s); tsp. = teaspoon(s).

Day 14

	1,700 Calories	1,900 Calories	2,100 Calories
Breakfast		*Western Omelet*	
		2 slices whole-wheat toast with	
		2 tsp. olive oil- or canola oil-based margarine	
		1½ cups skim milk	
Morning Snack	1 fresh peach	*Creamy Orange Shake*	
Lunch		1 serving of *Cheddar–Brazil Nut Salad*	
		1 cup skim milk	
Afternoon Snack	Tall glass of sugar-free iced tea		*Trail Mix I*
Dinner		4 oz. turkey breast	
		1 serving of *Cream Cheese Whipped Potatoes and Gravy*	
		1 cup green peas with 1 tsp. margarine	
		1 cup skim milk	
Evening Snack	*Creamy Orange Shake*		1 serving of *Strawberry Cheesecake*

Daily Nutrition Totals			
Calories	1,693	1,949	2,157
Protein (g)	123	138	143
Carbohydrates (g)	195	227	266
Fiber (g)	24	24	26
Fat (g)	48	56	62
% calories from fat	25	25	25
Distribution of fat type:			
Saturated	33%	36%	36%
Monounsaturated	44%	43%	42%
Polyunsaturated	23%	21%	22%
Vitamin B$_6$ (mg)	2.4	2.49	2.57
Folic acid (mcg)	488	516	541
Calcium (mg)	1,812	2,099	2,127
Iron (mg)	12	13	14
Zinc (mg)	13	13	14

g = gram(s); mcg = microgram(s); mg = milligram(s); oz. = ounce(s); tsp. = teaspoon(s).

THE MEAL PLAN: DOING IT YOURSELF

You have the option of following our meal plans, mixing and matching the meals to make a different set, or building your own set with the information we provide below. In case you want to design your own meals, we've divided up each set of calories into the number of servings you need from the different food groups. We've included two tables: one lists the total number of servings by food group and the other divides these servings into meals and snacks spread throughout the day. Of course, you can move the servings around to meet your own schedule, but do try to maintain some sense of balance, taking your cues from what we've done here and aiming for three meals and three snacks daily. For information on serving sizes and for more advice on creating your own meal plans, see Chapter Four.

Food Groups by Calorie Level

	1,700 Calories	1,900 Calories	2,100 Calories
Nonfat dairy	4 servings	4 servings	5 servings
Whole-grain foods	4 servings	5 servings	5 servings
Legumes	2 servings	2 servings	3 servings
Fruits	4 servings	4 servings	5 servings
Vegetables	5 servings	5 servings	5 servings
Lean protein	4 servings	4 servings	4 servings
Nuts or seeds	1.5 oz. nuts or 3 oz. seeds	2 oz. nuts or 4 oz. seeds	2 oz. nuts or 4 oz. seeds
Added fats	2 servings	3 servings	3 servings

oz. = ounces.

Food Groups by Meals and Calorie Levels

	1,700 Calories	1,900 Calories	2,100 Calories
Breakfast	1 milk 1 whole grain 1 fruit	1 milk 2 whole grains 2 fruits	1 milk 2 whole grains 2 fruits
Morning Snack	2 fruits	1 fruit	1 fruit
Lunch	1 milk 2 whole grains 2 legumes 3 vegetables	1 milk 2 whole grains 2 legumes 3 vegetables	1 milk 2 whole grains 3 legumes 3 vegetables
Afternoon Snack	1 milk 1 fruit	1 milk 1 fruit	1 milk 2 fruits
Dinner	1 whole grain 2 vegetables 4 lean proteins	1 whole grain 2 vegetables 4 lean proteins	1 whole grain 2 vegetables 4 lean proteins 1 milk

	1,700 Calories	*1,900 Calories*	*2,100 Calories*
Evening Snack	1 milk	1 milk	1 milk
	1.5 oz. nuts or	2 oz. nuts or	2 oz. nuts or
	3 oz. seeds	4 oz. seeds	4 oz. seeds
As Desired	2 servings	3 servings	3 servings
	added fats	added fats	added fats

oz. = ounces.

TROUBLESHOOTING

I'm Not Used to Eating Breakfast; How Can I Adjust?

Start small, such as with a small bowl of cereal or a yogurt. These foods are also easy and quick if you have little time in the morning. Remember, it is important to eat breakfast during pregnancy. Breakfast got its name because you are essentially breaking your overnight fast.

I Haven't Drunk Milk Since I Was a Kid; Why Can't I Wait until I Am Pregnant to Start Again?

Bones continue to grow in density until sometime in your twenties or thirties. So building up your bone density is exceptionally important, even if you were never even planning on having a baby. Doing so can prevent you from developing osteoporosis later in life. Now, as you await becoming pregnant, you can build up your bone density and form the storehouses that you and your baby will need. Also, it is good to start developing the habit now, before it becomes such a necessity.

I Am Lactose Intolerant and Have Never Been Able to Drink Milk; What Can I Do?

Now, fortunately, you have many choices to get the nutrients that milk provides. Just as an aside, milk is an important part of your diet for many reasons besides calcium: vitamin D, protein, and vitamin B_{12}. You can purchase Lactaid milk, or milk in which the lactose has already been broken down. Alternatively, you can treat the milk yourself, using drops available at your pharmacy. You can even treat yourself by taking a small tablet containing the enzyme lactase (also from your pharmacy) when you consume dairy products. Reduced-fat soy milk, now fortified with calcium and vitamins D and B_{12}, is also an option. If none of this works for you, use calcium–vitamin D supplements, checking with your physician regarding dosage.

CHAPTER SIX

The First-Trimester Optimal Diet

You're not alone if, during this first trimester, you are wondering what all the fuss is about. You're probably feeling fatigued, maybe nauseated, and most certainly are looking forward to feeling like your old self. Here, we'll give you some help in how to take in all the nutrition you and your baby need during this time when food can be anything but appetizing.

Keep it simple. Plan little for these first 3 months except time to take care of yourself. Work frequent naps into your daily routine or at least try to set aside some time to put up your feet at home and at work and some time to rest. Enjoy turning in early at night, using this wonderfully important excuse as one to get those 8 or so hours of sleep you need each night—the long night's sleep that you've only dreamed about in the past. If you have other children, go to bed when they do—don't worry about cleaning up toys and shining bathrooms. That can all wait until you are feeling better and more energetic.

Let's take a look at what is happening to you and baby during this time to build a good foundation of understanding your changing nutrition needs this trimester.

Mom's Changing Body

Month 1

In the first month of pregnancy, you will notice, as the first recognized sign of pregnancy, the absence of your menstrual period; in some cases, though, your period continues or you may just have spotting. You may also notice tingling, tender, or swollen breasts; nausea; minor uterine contractions; and fatigue. Many women feel a mix of emotions during the first months of pregnancy, ranging from excitement to fear, and experience an increase or decrease in appetite; you may also have cravings for food you don't normally eat. Although it is very early in your pregnancy, your growing uterus and placenta demand a good blood supply. This means that your body must begin producing more blood, a process that will continue throughout your pregnancy. Although these early blood-making demands are not great, they do increase your needs for certain nutrients so that you don't become anemic.

Month 2

By the second month, menstruation has usually ceased (if it has continued at all), but some women still have slight spotting. You may experience seemingly odd food cravings, morning sickness, heartburn, indigestion, flatulence, and breast tenderness. Because the uterus sits so low in the pelvic cavity right now, it crowds out the bladder, and you may feel the need for frequent urination. Generally, the food cravings don't tip your calorie intake over the edge because they are moderated by nausea and the other digestive issues you face, such as heartburn and indigestion—so give into your cravings and enjoy if they don't occur too frequently. Extra sleep or afternoon naps may be necessary to combat fatigue or sleepiness, and you may feel irritable and have mood swings. Your uterus and placenta are increasing in size, ever so slowly, which means that your body must continue to increase the amount of blood in your circulatory system.

Month 3

During the first trimester, morning sickness and strange food cravings are generally the most intense during the third month. In addition, you may experience frequent urination, constipation, slight headaches, dizziness, or skin problems such as rashes or acne. Constipation, which can be helped by dietary means, may become a significant issue at this stage of your pregnancy because the fetus still sits low in the pelvic area, resting on your intestinal tract and also on your bladder (which is why frequent urination continues to be a problem). You may continue to have mood swings between joy and anxiety. The ever-growing placenta and uterus, and now the baby's circulatory system, require continued blood volume expansion.

BABY'S CONSTRUCTION PROJECTS

Month 1

At the moment of conception, your child is a single cell. During the first month, the embryo is only the size of a pencil point, but already the vertebrae and jaw begin to develop. At just four weeks after conception, in fact, the brain and spinal column are completely formed. This early "construction" work requires sufficient amounts of folic acid, that notable nutrient of pregnancy you learned about earlier. It was only as recent as the 1990s that scientists have discovered that getting enough folic acid (also called folate) in the first few days of pregnancy may prevent most birth defects of the spinal column (also called neural tube defects), such as spina bifida. Tissues under construction also need several other nutrients, as we have outlined below in the "Nutrition Priorities" section.

Month 2

By the end of the second month, the embryo is about the size of a grain of rice and resembles a tadpole. Arm and leg buds are present, and eyes and ears begin to develop. The kidneys, heart, and other essential organs start to form during this month. As in month 1, you'll need to ensure that you get adequate amounts of the notable nutrients of pregnancy to support these ever-so-critical construction projects.

Month 3

Your child's heart will begin to beat during the third month, and her or his arms and legs will be formed, with tiny finger and toe buds. At 70 days after conception, the heart, kidneys, and other organs are completely formed and simply need to grow in size over the remainder of the pregnancy. At this point, your baby will weigh a scant .33 ounces and measure about 1.25 inches long. Although so tiny, your child-to-be demands the same critical "growing nutrients" that we've listed below under "Nutrition Priorities."

NUTRITION PRIORITIES

We've divided up the nutrition priorities of this trimester into the following categories:

- Getting enough calories for slow weight gain, as well as to prevent undernutrition and weight loss, and understanding how to cope with nausea
- Establishing the good habit of eating three meals and three snacks daily
- Obtaining enough folic acid to prevent neural tube defects and other birth defects
- Taking in adequate iron and all the nutrients that allow an increase in blood volume without causing anemia
- Consuming enough protein and the "growing nutrients" to support your baby's developing organs and tissues
- Stocking up on calcium

Getting the Right Amount of Calories for Slow Weight Gain

Try to at least maintain your weight during this trimester—and preferably to gain 3 to 5 pounds, especially if you were underweight before becoming pregnant. Preventing undernutrition (calorie and nutrientwise) may decrease your child-to-be's future risk of various diseases, including heart disease, obesity, high blood pressure, and diabetes mellitus. To help you maintain your weight, we recommend 1,900 or 2,200 calories. We don't list 1,700 calories here, as we do in the prepregnancy chapter, because that calorie level is too low during pregnancy.

We know, though, that eating right can be a real challenge during this first trimester, when you may be contending with morning sickness (or all-day queasiness) and food aversions. We're here to help! It may take a little experimenting to determine what you can eat during these early days of pregnancy, but we have some suggestions that we know work for many women:

- *Eat before you rise.* Some women find that nibbling on something even before they get out of bed in the morning is a tremendous help in preventing nausea. If your partner is home mornings, ask him or her to bring you breakfast in bed (maybe one of you can prepare it the night before and put it in the refrigerator). If that isn't possible, then store your breakfast in a small cooler next to your bed, just within reach. Finally, as one more option, select the very easy breakfast options at the end of this section, and simply place crispbread, whole-wheat pita bread, dry toast, or whole-wheat crackers next to your bed in a sealed container. If the worst thing you have to contend with is a few crumbs in bed, so be it!

- *Rise slowly.* Getting up slowly can help prevent that seasick feeling.
- *Don't get too hungry.* Many women find that hunger—even the slightest bit—leads to nausea. That's why we built in three snacks each day for this trimester. (As you'll see, we've actually included three snacks in each trimester, but for quite different reasons.) If you find that you need larger snacks than what we've included, then simply borrow some food from the meals to build larger snacks.
- *Take advantage of the best time.* Generally, you'll feel much more like eating at one time of the day than others. This time is indeed variable, but it is often in the late afternoon or evening. You may even find that this good time may vary from day to day. Whenever it is, take advantage of being nausea free and eat well. Some women find it helpful to prepare food for a whole day during their nausea-free period. On a particularly good day, you may want to cook ahead for several days that week.
- *Fill up your tank before bed.* Having a satisfying snack at bedtime can help prevent a truly empty feeling in the morning, which can lead to morning nausea.
- *Eat cold instead of hot.* Sometimes, sidestepping nausea is as easy as avoiding food smells. Something that smelled absolutely delicious before pregnancy may now be very offensive to you. One way to avoid the smell of food is to have cold meals (especially early in the day, or whenever your nausea is the worst) or to have someone else prepare your food. For example, you'll notice that we've included rotisserie chicken from the supermarket or deli in our meal plan. This way, you don't have to contend with the smell of cooking chicken, and you will also have leftovers for lunches and other meals. Investigate your supermarket and deli for other shortcuts.
- *Eat dry instead of wet.* The great majority of women find that dry food, such as crackers and bread, sits better in their stomach than more moist foods. If you are particularly troubled by nausea, find those dry food items that work for you (crispbread, toasted whole-wheat or rye bread, and so on).
- *Follow your stomach.* In other words, eat whatever tastes good to you. Although you might have loved salmon in your prepregnant days, now you might find it repulsive. Similarly, you may now crave potatoes or cheese or something else that might have seldom been a

part of your diet. We do recommend varying your diet (two fish meals, no more than two beef meals, no more than two poultry meals, and at least one vegetarian meal weekly for dinner), but we also acknowledge that your taste buds and your stomach are very fussy at this time. You should find the foods and recipes that are appealing to you and that keep your stomach on an even keel and use them frequently with your meal plans. We've provided a good deal of variety in the meals we've designed for this trimester, so we hope you'll find plenty that work for you. Do remember that what you loved yesterday may sound positively horrible today. That's entirely normal!

Establishing a Pattern of Eating Three Meals and Three Snacks Daily

In the best of all worlds, most people—pregnant or not—should divide up their daily calorie intake into three meals and three snacks. The advantage? When you eat this way, you give your body a "continuous feed" of energy. As you guessed, that can make you feel more energetic throughout the day, because your body never really runs on empty. Even during weight loss efforts, this is a great idea because you never truly become hungry, which can lead to bingeing.

During pregnancy, avoiding running on empty becomes even more important. After you eat a meal, your body digests, absorbs, and metabolizes the food, which provides a source of energy for your body. Eating several small meals provides a more constant stream of energy into your

Take Some Insurance

We agree with the latest official advice that you should harvest all of your nutrients during pregnancy from food rather than supplements, but we also know how difficult this is! Because this period of fetal development is so critically important and because there is strong possibility that you may not be able to take in a completely balanced diet during this first trimester, we highly recommend that you take a prenatal multivitamin and mineral supplement at this time. Ask your obstetrician or nurse midwife for the final word on this.

bloodstream than does eating just three larger meals. This is better to fuel your every activity and baby's needs, rather than having three large energy boosts throughout the day.

Obtaining Enough Folic Acid to Prevent Neural Tube Defects and Other Birth Defects

Of all the notable nutrients of pregnancy, folic acid stands at the head of the list. As we detailed earlier, folic acid may be the most important nutrient in terms of preventing birth defects. The discovery in the 1990s that folic acid may prevent spina bifida and other neural tube defects has been heralded as one of the most important medical discoveries of the twentieth century.

As we noted in Chapter Five, you should increase your folic acid intake when you are just thinking about becoming pregnant. This is because the most critical time to ensure adequate folic acid intake is in those very earliest days of pregnancy, often before you even know that you are pregnant.

Taking in Adequate Iron and Nutrients to Allow an Increase in Blood Volume Without Causing Anemia

During their reproductive years, women are vulnerable to anemia. This is because the iron lost via monthly menstruation can be difficult to replace by diet alone. Although menstruation ceases during pregnancy, women face another, greater, iron demand: getting enough iron to build the blood supply for the growing uterus, placenta, and the baby's circulation. Although iron needs don't increase from the prepregnancy requirement of 18 milligrams per day until about the twelfth week of pregnancy (when they rise to 30 milligrams daily), it is still important that women focus on getting enough iron early on. Doing so helps a woman build up a good level of iron stores, ready for the months ahead. As you can imagine, this is important in preventing iron-deficiency anemia when demands quickly increase as you approach the end of the third and the beginning of the fourth month.

In addition to iron, you'll need the other ingredients in the blood-building recipe. The nutrients that work with iron to make healthy red blood cells include copper, vitamin C, vitamin B_6, folic acid, vitamin B_{12}, and riboflavin.

Consuming Enough Protein and the "Growing Nutrients" to Support Your Baby's Developing Organs and Tissues

Protein provides the basis for the formation and growth of new tissues. To draw an analogy, flour is the basis, or main ingredient, of a loaf of bread. But just as that flour alone cannot make bread—it needs help from yeast, salt, a pinch of sugar, and some liquid—the protein alone cannot build your baby. Many nutrients contribute to this most important of recipes, but those of outstanding importance are zinc, vitamin B_6, and folic acid.

Stocking Up on Calcium

True, your baby's bones aren't yet big enough to demand any appreciable amounts of calcium. But Mother Nature was brilliant when she gave a mother-to-be's body the ability to absorb and then store increased amounts of calcium during the first trimester. This is very handy during the final trimester, when your baby's bones are growing rapidly and demanding so much calcium. So build up your calcium stores during this first trimester by enjoying plenty of calcium-rich foods.

Supplement Savvy

- Iron supplements may be particularly difficult to take when you are feeling nauseated during the first trimester. If you are anemic, ask your health-care provider about taking smaller doses of iron two to three times per day instead of one large dose. One other strategy: Take your iron just before bed (with your evening snack) so that you can sleep through any queasiness it may cause.
- If you do take iron (in any trimester), try to take it with foods rich in vitamin C. Vitamin C helps your body to absorb iron in supplements and also iron in foods of plant origin.
- When you must take calcium and iron supplements, take them at opposite times of the day (that is, if you take your calcium supplement in the morning, take your iron supplement at night). These nutrients compete with one another for absorption.
- Take any supplement with a meal or snack. Not only is absorption better but also, you'll avoid the stomach upset that many types of supplements can sometimes cause.

The First-Trimester Optimal Diet

To make your life easier, Kris Napier has designed two weeks of daily meal plans that take into account the special needs and feelings of women in their first trimester. Although the nutrient requirements are the same for the rest of the pregnancy, we've divided up the food slightly differently each trimester, depending on what is happening with you and your baby.

For instance, in this trimester, we've planned lighter, drier breakfasts to appease queasy stomachs. We've also planned a slightly heavier nighttime snack, as many women have an easier time eating at the end of the day than at the beginning. And, as we noted earlier in this chapter, eating a more substantial snack at night may keep your stomach from becoming so empty by morning—an emptiness that can lead to nausea.

Remember that each breakfast, lunch, and dinner in this trimester has the same calories as every other breakfast, lunch, and dinner. So, within each calorie level, you can enjoy any of the 14 breakfasts on any day during your first trimester (all at 300 calories each). Follow it up with any of the 14 lunches and dinners. (Each lunch for the 1,900- and 2,200-calorie levels has 450 calories and 550 calories, respectively. The dinners at both calorie levels have 550 calories.) Note that all meal plan items in italics signify recipes that you'll find in Chapter Ten.

Bon appetit!

Also to help queasy stomachs, we've designed several breakfasts, lunches, and dinners that definitely put you on dry land. Refer to the alternative meals listed after the meal plans for extra-easy-to-stomach menus for the worst of days. They may not provide a great deal of variety (so a multivitamin and mineral supplement is a wise idea), but they do contain enough of those critical calories.

Day 1

	1,900 Calories	2,200 Calories
Breakfast	1 poached egg	
	1 slice whole-wheat toast with 2 tsp. olive oil- or canola oil-based margarine	
	1 cup skim milk	
Morning Snack	1 cup Raisin Bran cereal with 1 tbsp. almonds and 1 cup skim milk	
Lunch	Peanut Butter Sandwich: 2 tbsp. natural peanut butter and 1 tbsp. jam or jelly on 2 slices whole-wheat bread 1 cup skim milk	Peanut Butter Sandwich: 3 tbsp. natural peanut butter and 1 tbsp. jam or jelly on 2 slices whole-wheat bread 1 cup skim milk
Afternoon Snack	¼ cup roasted sunflower seeds	¼ cup roasted sunflower seeds with 2 tbsp. raisins
Dinner	4 oz. skinless chicken breast (may purchase rotisserie chicken from supermarket)	
	1 baked sweet potato (about 4 oz. or 100 g) with 1 tbsp. margarine and 2 tsp. brown sugar	
Evening Snack	1 papaya (about 11 oz. or 300 g)	½ cup low-fat vanilla frozen yogurt with 1 papaya (about 11 oz. or 300 g)

Daily Nutrition Totals		
Calories	1,906	2,171
Protein (g)	110	119
Carbohydrates (g)	227	268
Fiber (g)	29	32
Fat (g)	71	81
% calories from fat	32	32
Distribution of fat type:		
Saturated	17%	20%
Monounsaturated	38%	34%
Polyunsaturated	45%	37%
Vitamin B$_6$ (mg)	2.88	3.04

Daily Nutrition Totals (continued)

Folic acid (mcg)	646	680
Calcium (mg)	1,500	1,669
Iron (mg)	34	36
Zinc (mg)	17	19

g = gram(s); mcg = microgram(s); mg = milligram(s); oz. = ounce(s); tbsp. = tablespoon(s); tsp. = teaspoons.

Day 2

	1,900 Calories	2,200 Calories
Breakfast	4 graham crackers with ½ cup extra-calcium low-fat cottage cheese	
	1 cup skim milk	
Morning Snack	1 cup Multi-grain Cheerios with 3 tbsp. dried cranberries (Craisins) and 1 cup skim milk	1 cup Multi-grain Cheerios with ¼ cup dried cranberries (Craisins) and 1 cup skim milk
Lunch	*Fresh 'n' Fruity Chicken Pasta*	*Fresh 'n' Fruity Chicken Pasta* 1 orange
Afternoon Snack	¼ cup dry roasted peanuts	
Dinner	Cheeseburger: 3-oz. hamburger patty, 1-oz. low-fat cheese, and 1 tomato slice on hamburger bun	
	Salad: 2 cups romaine lettuce, ¼ cup garbanzo beans, and 2 tomato slices with 2 tbsp. favorite low-fat salad dressing	
Evening Snack	2 cups fresh or frozen raspberries with 2 tbsp. low-fat frozen whipped topping	2 cups fresh or frozen raspberries with ¼ cup low-fat frozen whipped topping and 2 tbsp. almonds

Daily Nutrition Totals

Calories	1,933	2,140
Protein (g)	124	128
Carbohydrates (g)	248	276
Fiber (g)	39	45

Fat (g)	54	64
% calories from fat	25	26
Distribution of fat type:		
Saturated	29%	29%
Monounsaturated	42%	46%
Polyunsaturated	29%	25%
Vitamin B$_6$ (mg)	2.22	2.31
Folic acid (mcg)	800	851
Calcium (mg)	1,433	1,534
Iron (mg)	24	25
Zinc (mg)	18	18

g = gram(s); mcg = microgram(s); mg = milligram(s); oz. = ounce(s);
tbsp. = tablespoon(s).

Day 3		
	1,900 Calories	***2,200 Calories***
Breakfast	1 cup mandarin orange sections, fresh or canned in juice	
	1 cup low-fat lemon yogurt	
Morning Snack	1 small plain bagel	1 small plain bagel, 1 cup skim milk
Lunch	Grilled Cheese Sandwich: 3 oz. low-fat cheese on 2 slices whole wheat bread with 2 tbsp. margarine	Grilled Cheese Sandwich: 3 oz. low-fat cheese on 2 slices whole-wheat bread with 2 tbsp. olive oil- or canola oil-based margarine
	1 banana	1 banana
		1 cup skim milk
Afternoon Snack	1 cup low-fat fruit yogurt	
Dinner	4 oz. beef tenderloin	
	1 baked potato (about 7 oz. or 200 g) with 2 tbsp. low-fat sour cream	
	1 cup steamed green beans with 1 tbsp. almonds	

Day 3 (*continued*)

	1,900 Calories	2,200 Calories
Evening Snack	½ cup roasted pumpkin seeds	½ cup roasted pumpkin seeds, 1 cup calcium-fortified orange juice

Daily Nutrition Totals		
Calories	1,919	2,210
Protein (g)	98	115
Carbohydrates (g)	278	329
Fiber (g)	27	27
Fat (g)	51	52
% calories from fat	23	21
Distribution of fat type:		
Saturated	48%	47%
Monounsaturated	33%	32%
Polyunsaturated	19%	21%
Vitamin B$_6$ (mg)	1.76	2.08
Folic acid (mcg)	464	534
Calcium (mg)	2,101	3004
Iron (mg)	12	12
Zinc (mg)	16	18

g = gram(s); mcg = microgram(s); mg = milligram(s); oz. = ounce(s);
tbsp. = tablespoon(s).

Day 4

	1,900 Calories	2,200 Calories
Breakfast	1 *Cranberry Pumpkin Muffin*	
	1 cup skim milk	
Morning Snack	*Trail Mix I*	*Trail Mix I,* 1½ cups calcium-fortified orange juice
Lunch	Turkey–Spinach Pita: 3 oz. skinless turkey breast, 2 cups chopped spinach (or bagged baby spinach), and 2 tbsp. favorite low-fat salad dressing in 1 whole-wheat pita	Turkey–Spinach Pita: 3 oz. skinless turkey breast, 2 cups chopped spinach (or bagged baby spinach), and 2 tbsp. favorite low-fat salad dressing in 1 whole-wheat pita

	1,900 Calories	**2,200 Calories**
Lunch (*cont.*)	1 cup skim milk	1 cup skim milk
		1 fresh peached, sliced, with 2 tbsp. low-fat frozen whipped topping and 1 tbsp. almonds
Afternoon Snack	7 vanilla wafers, 1 cup skim milk	
Dinner	*Easy Cheesy Pasta Salad*	
	2 cups broccoli with ¼ cup fat-free sour cream	
Evening Snack	*Chocolate Shake*	

Daily Nutrition Totals		
Calories	1,885	2,168
Protein (g)	110	112
Carbohydrates (g)	290	343
Fiber (g)	23	26
Fat (g)	37	43
% calories from fat	17	17
Distribution of fat type:		
Saturated	40%	37%
Monounsaturated	40%	44%
Polyunsaturated	20%	19%
Vitamin B$_6$ (mg)	2.38	2.58
Folic acid (mcg)	326	399
Calcium (mg)	1,414	1,868
Iron (mg)	17	18
Zinc (mg)	14	15

g = gram(s); mcg = microgram(s); mg = milligram(s); oz. = ounce(s); tbsp. = tablespoon(s).

Day 5		
	1,900 Calories	*2,200 Calories*
Breakfast	1 cup low-fat vanilla yogurt with 1 banana, sliced	
Morning Snack	½ small plain bagel	½ small plain bagel with 1 tbsp. natural peanut butter, 1 cup skim milk
Lunch	1 serving of *Rainbow Meal Salad*	1 serving of *Rainbow Meal Salad*
	½ cup skim milk	1 cup skim milk
		1 favorite flavor Newton cookie
Afternoon Snack	1 papaya (about 11 oz. or 300 g)	
Dinner	1 serving of *Cheesy Spinach Pizza*	
	½ cup calcium-fortified orange juice	
Evening Snack	*Banana Split*	

Daily Nutrition Totals		
Calories	1,958	2,239
Protein (g)	80	98
Carbohydrates (g)	312	343
Fiber (g)	39	41
Fat (g)	52	62
% calories from fat	23	24
Distribution of fat type:		
Saturated	40%	36%
Monounsaturated	40%	41%
Polyunsaturated	20%	23%
Vitamin B$_6$ (mg)	2.82	3.03
Folic acid (mcg)	844	887
Calcium (mg)	1,602	2,063
Iron (mg)	178	19
Zinc (mg)	9	11

g = gram(s); mcg = microgram(s); mg = milligram(s); oz. = ounce(s); tbsp. = tablespoon(s).

Day 6

	1,900 Calories	*2,200 Calories*
Breakfast	*Peach Shake* 1 hard-boiled egg	
Morning Snack	1 slice whole-wheat toast with 2 tsp. jam or jelly	1 slice whole-wheat toast with 2 tsp. jam or jelly, 1½ cups skim milk
Lunch	*Sweet Walnut Wrap*	*Sweet Walnut Wrap*
	½ cup skim milk	1½ cups skim milk
Afternoon Snack	2 cups broccoli and 1 red bell pepper, sliced, with ¼ cup fat-free sour cream for dip	2 cups broccoli and 1 red bell pepper, sliced, with ¼ cup fat-free sour cream for dip; ½ cup calcium-fortified orange juice
Dinner	1 serving of *Cream Cheese Whipped Potatoes and Gravy*	
	One 4-oz. pork chop	
	6 steamed asparagus spears	
	1 cup skim milk	
	1 fresh orange	
Evening Snack	1 *Banana Chocolate Chip Muffin*	1 *Banana Chocolate Chip Muffin*, ½ cup skim milk

Daily Nutrition Totals		
Calories	1,832	2,172
Protein (g)	113	136
Carbohydrates (g)	270	326
Fiber (g)	32	32
Fat (g)	42	43
% calories from fat	20	17
Distribution of fat type:		
Saturated	53%	54%
Monounsaturated	34%	31%
Polyunsaturated	13%	15%

Daily Nutrition Totals (continued)		
Vitamin B$_6$ (mg)	2.42	2.82
Folic acid (mcg)	663	749
Calcium (mg)	1,714	2,833
Iron (mg)	13	14
Zinc (mg)	11	14

g = gram(s); mcg = microgram(s); mg = milligram(s); oz. = ounce(s);
tsp. = teaspoon(s).

Day 7

	1,900 Calories	2,200 Calories
Breakfast	1 cup extra-calcium low-fat cottage cheese with 1 whole-wheat pita pocket	
Morning Snack	2 cups favorite dry cereal	2 cups favorite dry cereal with 1½ cups skim milk
Lunch	*Hummus Wrap*	*Hummus Wrap*
	1 cup skim milk	1 cup skim milk
	1 cup fresh or frozen raspberries	2 cups fresh or frozen raspberries
Afternoon Snack	¼ cup walnuts	
Dinner	4 oz. skinless chicken breast, grilled	
	1 serving of *Lemon-Fresh Rotini Spinach*	
	1 cup skim milk	
Evening Snack	1 cup sliced strawberries with ½ cup vanilla ice cream	1 cup sliced strawberries with ¾ cup vanilla ice cream

Daily Nutrition Totals		
Calories	1,929	2,175
Protein (g)	126	140
Carbohydrates (g)	248	287
Fiber (g)	41	50
Fat (g)	59	64
% calories from fat	26	25

Distribution of fat type:

Saturated	38%	37%
Monounsaturated	43%	42%
Polyunsaturated	19%	21%
Vitamin B$_6$ (mg)	3.1	3.32
Folic acid (mcg)	976	1,027
Calcium (mg)	1,607	2,095
Iron (mg)	33	34
Zinc (mg)	18	20

g = gram(s); mcg = microgram(s); mg = milligram(s); oz. = ounce(s).

Day 8	
1,900 Calories	**2,200 Calories**

Breakfast	2 oat bran waffles	
	1 cup skim milk	
Morning Snack	1 serving of *Ready-to-go Fruit Salad*	1 serving of *Ready-to-go Fruit Salad* with 2 tbsp. dry-roasted peanuts
Lunch	Tossed Rotini with Broccoli: 1 cup cooked rotini pasta tossed with 1 tsp. extra-virgin olive oil, ¼ cup grated parmesan cheese, and 2 cups steamed broccoli	Tossed Rotini with Broccoli: 1 cup cooked rotini pasta tossed with 1 tsp. extra-virgin olive oil, ¼ cup grated parmesan cheese, and 2 cups steamed broccoli
		1 cup skim milk
Afternoon Snack	½ small plain bagel with 2 oz. roast beef and 1 cup romaine lettuce	1 small plain bagel with 2 oz. roast beef and 1 cup romaine lettuce
Dinner	1 serving of *Orange–Spinach Salad*	
	1 serving of *Scalloped Potatoes*	
Evening Snack	*Creamy Orange Shake*	

Daily Nutrition Totals		
Calories	1,910	2,200
Protein (g)	109	125
Carbohydrates (g)	256	291
Fiber (g)	34	36
Fat (g)	54	64
% calories from fat	25	26
Distribution of fat type:		
Saturated	26%	26%
Monounsaturated	44%	44%
Polyunsaturated	30%	30%
Vitamin B$_6$ (mg)	2.49	2.66
Folic acid (mcg)	1,119	1,189
Calcium (mg)	1,860	2,197
Iron (mg)	18	21
Zinc (mg)	13	15

g = gram(s); mcg = microgram(s); mg = milligram(s); oz. = ounce(s);
tsp. = teaspoon(s).

Day 9		
	1,900 Calories	**2,200 Calories**
Breakfast	*Cheesy Mushroom Omelet*	
	½ small plain bagel with 1 tsp. margarine	
	½ cup skim milk	
Morning Snack	¼ of a honeydew melon	
Lunch	Roast Beef Sandwich: 3 oz. roast beef, 2 tsp. light mayonnaise, and 1 cup baby spinach on 2 slices whole-wheat bread	Roast Beef Sandwich: 3 oz. roast beef, 2 tsp. light mayonnaise, and 1 cup baby spinach on 2 slices whole-wheat bread
	1 cup skim milk 1 orange	1 cup skim milk 1 orange 1 favorite flavor Newton cookie
Afternoon Snack	*Trail Mix I*	2 servings of *Trail Mix I*

	1,900 Calories	2,200 Calories
Dinner	1 serving of *Taste of Summer Vegetable Lentil Soup*	
	1 serving of *Simple Garden Salad*	
	1 cup skim milk	
Evening Snack	*Frozen Lemonade*	

Daily Nutrition Totals		
Calories	1,904	2,233
Protein (g)	115	122
Carbohydrates (g)	290	349
Fiber (g)	43	47
Fat (g)	39	48
% calories from fat	18	19
Distribution of fat type:		
Saturated	23%	29%
Monounsaturated	50%	54%
Polyunsaturated	23%	21%
Vitamin B$_6$ (mg)	2.24	2.33
Folic acid (mcg)	800	824
Calcium (mg)	1,618	1,646
Iron (mg)	18	20
Zinc (mg)	13	14

g = gram(s); mcg = microgram(s); mg = milligram(s); oz. = ounce(s);
tsp. = teaspoon(s).

Day 10		
	1,900 Calories	**2,200 Calories**
Breakfast	2 slices whole-wheat toast with 4 tsp. jam or jelly	
	1 cup skim milk	
Morning Snack	¼ cup roasted sunflower seeds	¼ cup roasted sunflower seeds with ¼ cup raisins

Day 10 *(continued)*

	1,900 Calories	*2,200 Calories*
Lunch	*Black Bean Avocado Wrap*	*Black Bean Avocado Wrap*
	1 cup skim milk	1½ cups skim milk
	1 fresh orange	1 cup grapes
Afternoon Snack	*Double Raspberry Shake*	
Dinner	1 serving of *Roasted Chicken and Veggies*	
	½ cup skim milk	
Evening Snack	½ cup vanilla ice cream	1 cup vanilla ice cream with 1 peach, sliced

Daily Nutrition Totals		
Calories	1,871	2,255
Protein (g)	108	116
Carbohydrates (g)	298	375
Fiber (g)	48	50
Fat (g)	42	51
% calories from fat	19	19
Distribution of fat type:		
Saturated	28%	35%
Monounsaturated	33%	30%
Polyunsaturated	39%	35%
Vitamin B$_6$ (mg)	2.37	2.66
Folic acid (mcg)	425	405
Calcium (mg)	1,516	1,708
Iron (mg)	16	17
Zinc (mg)	11	13

g = gram(s); mcg = microgram(s); mg = milligram(s); oz. = ounce(s);
tsp. = teaspoon(s).

Day 11

	1,900 Calories	*2,200 Calories*
Breakfast	2 poached eggs	
	1 whole-wheat pita pocket	
Morning Snack	1½ cups Total cereal with ¾ cup skim milk	
Lunch	1 small whole-wheat bagel 1 cup extra-calcium low-fat cottage cheese	1 small whole-wheat bagel 1 cup extra-calcium low-fat cottage cheese
	1 pear	1 pear
	½ cup skim milk	1½ cups skim milk
Afternoon Snack	1 fresh orange	*Trail Mix III,* ½ cup skim milk
Dinner	Grilled Ham and Cheese: 2 oz. lean ham and 1 oz. low-fat cheddar cheese on 2 slices whole-wheat bread with 2 tsp. margarine	
	1 serving of *Salad of Many Greens (Side)*	
	½ cup skim milk	
Evening Snack	1 serving of *Orange Cream Fruit Tart*	

Daily Nutrition Totals		
Calories	1,927	2,191
Protein (g)	105	120
Carbohydrates (g)	262	299
Fiber (g)	34	37
Fat (g)	58	68
% calories from fat	26	27
Distribution of fat type:		
Saturated	26%	25%
Monounsaturated	52%	59%
Polyunsaturated	22%	21%
Vitamin B$_6$ (mg)	4.79	5.12
Folic acid (mcg)	1,227	1,266

Daily Nutrition Totals (*continued*)		
Calcium (mg)	1,815	2,237
Iron (mg)	44	48
Zinc (mg)	13	14

g = gram(s); mcg = microgram(s); mg = milligram(s); tsp. = teaspoon(s).

Day 12

	1,900 Calories	**2,200 Calories**
Breakfast	1 slice whole-wheat toast with 1 tbsp. natural peanut butter and 1 tbsp. jam or jelly	
	1 cup skim milk	
Morning Snack	1 Nutri-Grain cereal bar, 1 cup skim milk	1 Nutri-Grain cereal bar, 1½ cups skim milk
Lunch	1 serving of *Taste of Summer Lentil Vegetable Soup*	1 serving of *Taste of Summer Lentil Vegetable Soup*
	½ whole-wheat pita pocket	1 whole-wheat pita pocket
	½ cup skim milk	½ cup skim milk
Afternoon Snack	*Veggie Salsa Snack*	
Dinner	*Sweet and Sour Salmon Steaks*	
Evening Snack	1 cup low-fat frozen yogurt with 2 tbsp. light chocolate syrup	1 cup low-fat frozen yogurt with 2 tbsp. light chocolate syrup and 2 tbsp. dry-roasted peanuts

Daily Nutrition Totals		
Calories	1,936	2,161
Protein (g)	113	125
Carbohydrates (g)	307	333
Fiber (g)	40	44
Fat (g)	36	46
% calories from fat	16	18

Distribution of fat type:

Saturated	27%	23%
Monounsaturated	53%	53%
Polyunsaturated	20%	24%
Vitamin B$_6$ (mg)	4.17	4.34
Folic acid (mcg)	682	729
Calcium (mg)	1,662	1,754
Iron (mg)	20	22
Zinc (mg)	13	15

g = gram(s); mcg = microgram(s); mg = milligram(s); oz. = ounce(s);
tbsp. = tablespoon(s).

Day 13

	1,900 Calories	2,200 Calories
Breakfast	1 whole-wheat pita pocket with 2 tsp. jam or jelly	
	1 cup skim milk	
Morning Snack	1 papaya (about 11 oz. or 300 g)	
Lunch	2 cups low-sodium chicken noodle soup	2 cups low-sodium chicken noodle soup
	6 whole-wheat crackers with 2 oz. favorite reduced-fat cheese	6 whole-wheat crackers with 2 oz. favorite reduced-fat cheese
	½ cup skim milk	½ cup skim milk
		2 kiwis
Afternoon Snack	¼ cup roasted sunflower seeds with ¼ cup dried cranberries (Craisins)	½ cup roasted sunflower seeds with ¼ cup dried cranberries (Craisins)
Dinner	1 serving of *Poppyseed Salmon Salad*	
	4 whole-wheat crackers	
	Frozen Lemonade	
Evening Snack	2 whole-grain waffles	

Daily Nutrition Totals		
Calories	1,934	2,256
Protein (g)	110	122
Carbohydrates (g)	261	297
Fiber (g)	26	35
Fat (g)	57	74
% calories from fat	26	28
Distribution of fat type:		
Saturated	32%	28%
Monounsaturated	27%	24%
Polyunsaturated	41%	48%
Vitamin B$_6$ (mg)	1.75	2.15
Folic acid (mcg)	628	726
Calcium (mg)	1,615	1,827
Iron (mg)	14	15
Zinc (mg)	9	12

g = gram(s); mcg = microgram(s); mg = milligram(s); oz. = ounce(s);
tsp. = teaspoon(s).

Day 14		
	1,900 Calories	*2,200 Calories*
Breakfast	1 toasted English muffin with 2 oz. favorite reduced-fat cheese	
	1 kiwi	
Morning Snack	*Peanut Butter–Chocolate Shake*	
Lunch	*Veggie Pita*	*Veggie Pita*
	1 cup skim milk	1 cup skim milk
		1 apple
Afternoon Snack	½ cup fresh or frozen raspberries with 1 cup low-fat vanilla yogurt	1 cup fresh or frozen raspberries with 1 cup low-fat vanilla yogurt
Dinner	1 serving of *Legal Fettuccine Alfredo*	
	½ cup steamed peas	
Evening Snack	2 oz. oat bran pretzels	

Daily Nutrition Totals		
Calories	1,970	2,156
Protein (g)	94	100
Carbohydrates (g)	313	351
Fiber (g)	46	50
Fat (g)	45	47
% calories from fat	20	19
Distribution of fat type:		
Saturated	37%	40%
Monounsaturated	38%	40%
Polyunsaturated	25%	20%
Vitamin B$_6$ (mg)	1.25	1.38
Folic acid (mcg)	408	425
Calcium (mg)	1,222	1,441
Iron (mg)	13	13
Zinc (mg)	8	9

g = gram(s); mcg = microgram(s); mg = milligram(s); oz. = ounce(s).

Alternative Breakfasts

12 whole wheat crackers
1 cup skim milk
  or
2 whole-wheat pita pockets
  or
4 slices whole-wheat toast
  or
12 slices of crispbread

Alternative Lunches

Note: If you're following the 1,900-calorie plan, omit the food in brackets.

1 baked potato (about 7 ounces or 200 grams) with 3 ounces reduced-fat cheddar cheese and 2 tablespoons fat-free sour cream
[1 cup skim milk]
  or

2 servings of *Cream Cheese Whipped Potatoes and Gravy*
2 ounces favorite low-fat cheese
1 cup skim milk
[1 cup grapes]
   or
1½ cups favorite dry cereal with 1 cup skim milk
2 ounces favorite cheese
[1 banana]

Alternative Dinners

20 whole-wheat crackers
1½ cups skim milk
   or
2 whole-wheat pita pockets
1½ cups skim milk
   or
3½ cups corn flakes with 1½ cups skim milk

THE MEAL PLAN: DOING IT YOURSELF

We do know that there may be days when you don't want to follow our meal plans or eat the alternative meals provided. On these days, you can design your own meal plans by using the table "Food Groups by Calorie Level" and referring to the tables on pages 94 through 96 for serving sizes of food. We suggest that you use the table "Food Groups by Meals" to divide your food servings into meals and snacks, but you can eat the food servings whenever you wish.

Food Groups by Calorie Level

	1,900 Calories	*2,200 Calories*
Nonfat dairy	4 servings	5 servings
Whole-grain foods	6 servings	7 servings
Legumes	2 servings	3 servings
Fruits	3 servings	4 servings
Vegetable	5 servings	5 servings
Lean proteins	4 servings	4 servings
Nuts or seeds	2 oz. nuts or 4 oz. seeds	2 oz. nuts or 4 oz. seeds
Added fat	2 servings	3 servings

oz. = ounce(s).

Food Groups by Meals

	1,900 Calories	*2,200 Calories*
Breakfast	2 whole grains 1 lean protein	2 whole grains 1 lean protein
Morning Snack	1 milk 1 whole grain	2 milk 2 whole grains
Lunch	2 whole grains 1 fruit 2 vegetables 2 legumes	2 whole grains 1 fruit 2 vegetables 3 legumes
Afternoon Snack	2 fruits 1 milk	2 fruits 1 milk
Dinner	3 lean proteins 1 whole grain 1 milk 3 vegetables	3 lean proteins 1 whole grain 1 milk 3 vegetables
Evening Snack	1 fruit 1 milk 2 oz. nuts or 4 oz. seeds	2 fruits 1 milk 2 oz. nuts or 4 oz. seeds
As Desired	2 servings added fat	2 servings added fat

oz. = ounce(s).

Just as we provided a list of breakfasts for those especially queasy days, we have also developed a list that lets you develop meals from just a few food groups: breads, lean protein, and good fats. Of course, this is not an optimal way to eat, but these meal guidelines can be incredibly useful on days when you are very queasy. Dry whole-grain foods (crispbread, whole-wheat pita bread, brown rice, pasta, whole-wheat crackers, and soda crackers) and cold high-protein foods will get you through the day, and you'll also be assured of having enough calories. To reiterate what we said earlier in this chapter, it's wise to take a vitamin–mineral supplement if nausea forces you to eat this way. Just take it with food before bed to reduce the chances that it will cause more nausea. (If you have diabetes, seek your doctor's advice on how to handle nausea rather than following this plan.)

Food Servings in Starches and Lean Protein

	1,900 Calories	*2,200 Calories*
Whole-Grain Foods	12 servings	14 servings
Lean Protein	10 oz.	10 oz.
Olive Oil- or Canola-Based Margarine	2 tsp.	4 tsp.

oz. = ounce(s); tsp. = teaspoon(s).

TROUBLESHOOTING

I Simply Cannot Stand the Thought of Eating in the Morning; What Can I Do?

Try three things: first, eat a hearty snack at night before you go to bed. This will help prevent you from getting overly hungry overnight, a factor that can trigger nausea in the morning. Next, place a container of crackers or bread next to your bed and have a portion before rising. Wait a while after eating, then, rise slowly and begin your day, in slow motion so to speak. Crispbread is a great example of a food you may want to use. Contrary to many types of crackers, which can be loaded with hydrogenated fats, crispbread is virtually fat free, yet it still has a satisfying crunch.

Can I Have Caffeine-Containing Beverages?

It is best to give up all caffeine-containing beverages when you are thinking about becoming pregnant, or certainly as soon as you know you are. Many people who give up coffee and other caffeine-containing beverages quickly tend to have caffeine withdrawal headaches. To prevent this, wean yourself from coffee, tea, and other beverages over a couple of days.

I've Never Been a Breakfast Eater; Must I Eat Breakfast Now?

Absolutely yes! You and your baby have lots of construction projects going on every millisecond of the day. Try some of the plainer, easier breakfasts if you don't have time to make a big fuss.

I've Never Used Black Beans or Lentils Before; Must I Start Including These Things in My Diet?

There are no musts in our recommendations. If there is a food you simply don't like, you don't have to force yourself to eat it. As we've mentioned throughout this book, our goal is to help you eat healthier now and throughout your life. We are thinking about a lifetime of good health, not just your time during pregnancy. Learning how to include vegetable sources of protein, such as black beans, lentils, and garbanzo beans, is advisable to help you harvest the optimal proportion of nutrients every day and to help prevent chronic illnesses. Just give it a try—you may like it!

Since I've Started Eating More Whole Grains and Legumes, I Have More Intestinal Gas Than Usual; Is It the Fiber?

This is very possible. You need the amount of fiber we designed into the meal plans, but it does take a little time to get used to it. The average American eats only about 15 grams of fiber per day, when 25 is the recommended minimum. If you are having a lot of trouble with gas and bloating, then cut back on these foods and add them in a little more gradually. For example, if we've called for 1 cup of brown rice somewhere, mix ½ cup of brown rice and ½ cup of white rice, and then gradually increase the proportion of brown rice.

I Am So Tired Now That I Really Don't Want to Cook; Can I Make a Large Batch of Something in the Recipes and Then Eat the Same Thing for a Couple of Days?

Certainly you can. Ideally, you should eat a variety of different foods every day, but we know this isn't always possible, especially now when you are so fatigued. So do make a batch of something you like from our meal plans and then round it out with the other foods listed on the menu. That way, you may be able to cook just two or three times per week and then use leftovers the rest of the week. When you are feeling better, you can add more variety into your diet. In the meantime, however, a multivitamin and mineral supplement can help to ensure an adequate nutrient intake.

CHAPTER SEVEN

The Second-Trimester Optimal Diet

Don't feel you are unusual if you can summarize your feelings in the word *hungry*! For many women, it seems as though someone simply flipped a switch around week 13 or 14 and caused them to go from queasy to ravenously hungry. For other women, the transition may be more gradual. The queasiness of the first trimester may start easing up a meal here and then a day there.

In addition, the hormonal milieu of the second trimester tends to grant most women newfound energy. That nagging fatigue of the first trimester gradually lifts, uncovering a wonderful, almost magical, amount of energy. The developing baby isn't very big, so he or she doesn't seem like such a heavy load yet.

When feeling better, many women face a problem opposite to the one they had in the first trimester. Rather than asking, "How can I possibly eat?" many moms-to-be now worry how they'll avoid burglarizing the ice cream truck!

To the rescue! The advice in this chapter, the meal plans, and the recipes Kris Napier has developed for you will keep you on track, I promise! Kris has built in something of a treat every day. Don't worry, though; each of these treats has plenty of the nutrients (and even extra!) that you and your baby crave.

Mom's Changing Body

Month 4

During the fourth month, you will probably continue to experience morning sickness, breast tenderness, and other symptoms. But the nausea will abate and you may begin to experience food cravings and an increased appetite. You may continue to have mood swings, but these, too, will even out. Your sleep may continue to be disrupted by frequent urination, but this, too, will abate. During this time, your blood volume continues to increase, to an even greater extent, which stresses your body nutritionally.

Month 5

Morning sickness has usually subsided by the fifth month of pregnancy, leading to an increased appetite, and the increased urination frequency you've been experiencing may cease entirely, bringing urination back to normal. You typically feel more energetic and excited. The pregnancy is now starting to show, and you may begin to feel your baby move. Some women begin to experience nasal congestion, nosebleeds, hemorrhoids, white vaginal discharge, and mild ankle swelling. This is often the time that many women first develop iron-deficiency anemia without proper nutrition.

Month 6

By the sixth month, you will feel distinct fetal movement. You may begin to experience lower abdominal aches, backache, leg cramps, increased pulse, skin changes, heartburn, indigestion, and bloating, especially toward the end of this month. You will have fewer mood swings but occasional absentmindedness and irritability. Food cravings continue to be a problem. As your baby grows—and you along with him or her—you may need to change sleeping positions so that you don't feel like you are sleeping on a watermelon. This can lead to loss of sleep and then fatigue.

As you approach the third trimester, the metabolic milieu of pregnancy can begin to affect your body's ability to metabolize carbohydrates, and some women's blood sugars may begin to rise. Changes during pregnancy lead a small number of women to develop a special type of diabetes called gestational diabetes. Because diabetes must be particularly strictly controlled during pregnancy to avoid affecting the baby, it is very important that all pregnant women are tested for it sometime during the fifth or sixth month of pregnancy. Be sure to ask your physician or midwife about this if he or she doesn't bring it up. You can read more about this condition in Chapter Nine.

BABY'S CONSTRUCTION PROJECTS

Month 4

At the fourth month, your baby will be approximately 2½ to 3 inches long, with a disproportionately large head, and will weigh about ½ ounce. By the end of the fourth month, the eyes and ears will be fully developed, and most major organs, the circulatory system, and the urinary tract are operating. Although "construction nutrients" aren't as important to prevent developmental abnormalities or birth defects, they now become important to support tissue growth.

Month 5

At the halfway point in your pregnancy, your baby will be about 4 inches long, with well-defined fingers and toes. Tooth buds appear, and you may begin to feel the baby moving.

Month 6

Your baby will be about 8 to 10 inches long at the end of the second trimester and will be covered with protective soft down. Hair will begin to grow on the baby's head, and white eyelashes will appear. Your baby is developed enough to have the possibility of survival outside the womb in a hospital intensive care unit. Growth rate quickens, and that means your baby needs a sure, steady intake of protein, as well as the other notable nutrients.

NUTRITION PRIORITIES

- Avoid overnutrition while eating all the calories you and your baby need every day
- Focus on iron intake and avoid anemia
- Include foods rich in all the notable nutrients of pregnancy

Avoid Overnutrition

The transition from first to second trimester brings a lot of changes in your and your baby's growing bodies, which translates into different nutrition priorities for this trimester. In the first trimester, our goal was to avoid undernutrition; however, now we shift to avoiding overnutrition. Of course, you still need to take in an adequate number of calories and all the necessary vitamins and minerals, but as your appetite increases during this trimester, you are much more likely to take in too many calories than too few. As you would realize, this may lead to an overly large, heavy baby, which, in turn, may be associated with an increased risk for breast cancer and weight problems for the baby in its adult years.

Even though we covered the details of serving size in Chapter Four, we'd just like to reiterate how important it is to pay attention to these serving sizes now. When you are particularly hungry, you may be tempted not to measure and to just let your eyes be your guide. But when your appetite is in overdrive, it is even more important that you measure, especially when you are making the treats and shakes that we've designed into your menus. Here are a few more ways to control your portion and your appetite.

Eat an Especially Filling Breakfast
Yes, we're going to make you proactive in fighting off those ravenous food fantasies! Pleasing and nourishing your body at the beginning of the day is one beneficial way to do this. You'll find our breakfast dishes filling, fun, and delicious—a great way to be less hungry during the day.

Have Three Meals and Three Snacks Daily
Just when you think about eating will be the time that we want you to eat! That's why the three snacks and three regular meals are so important. We hope it will be harder to get hungry when your fuel tank is never really empty. We've indicated that you should eat specific snacks at certain times of the day, but please plan them according to your own appetite. If you have a chocolate shake on the menu one day after your evening meal but you want it for your 10:30 A.M. snack, go for it! You have the flexibility to have whatever size snack that is planned for that day whenever you need it.

Plan on Something Fabulous Tasting Every Day
Planning on a great-tasting shake, muffin, or brownie every day is a wonderful way not to crave treats. Just like eating a good breakfast, this is a

way of proactively eating less. Without this book, I agree you'd have a hard time doing this and still having enough calories for the nutrients you need *and* staying within the recommended number of calories that will help ensure just the right weight gain. But take a look (right now!) at the list of desserts, shakes, and smoothies (page 324) Kris Napier developed with an eye to your nutrition. Also, check out the list of muffins, breads, and cereals (page 220). I promise you'll love everything—even with all those terribly nutritious ingredients they call for. Whoever thought satisfying your sweet tooth would mean loading up on folic acid and calcium? (See Orange Cream Fruit Tart on page 327.)

Focus on Iron Intake and Avoid Anemia

Of the notable nutrients, iron takes precedence in the second trimester. Your body's increased need for this mineral means that anemia, caused by low iron stores in your body, becomes a greater risk and that you are more likely to require an iron supplement. Sometime during this trimester, many women find that their blood counts (hemoglobin and hematocrit, two measures of the amount of iron in your blood) drop. This happens because the baby demands much more iron as pregnancy proceeds (as you can see from "Baby's Construction Projects," your baby begins to grow much more quickly during this trimester) and also because your body has somewhat of a delayed reaction to the fact that your body began producing extra blood to supply the baby and placenta in the first trimester.

Although you might not have been taking iron supplements in the early stages of pregnancy, you may need them now. It is the rare woman who can take in enough iron through food alone to meet these demands, so don't feel bad if you need to take a supplement. We have built in as much iron as we possibly can in dietary form, but do take the supplement if your obstetrician or nurse midwife says you need it. Make sure you have monthly blood tests to check on your blood counts.

One note on food sources of iron: When eating plant foods that are rich in iron, such as greens, whole-grain foods, and legumes, have a food rich in vitamin C at the same meal or snack. Meat sources of iron are often readily absorbed on their own, but plant sources need a little help, which vitamin C provides. Think of the vitamin C as the carrier. These foods, including citrus fruits or juices, berries, melon, tomatoes, and peppers, will help your body absorb more of the plant-based iron.

Include Foods Rich in All the Notable Nutrients of Pregnancy

Although the body doesn't need any more of the other notable nutrients than it did during the first trimester, they are all still quintessentially important in your baby's development. For example, calcium is required for your baby's developing skeleton and tooth buds, and protein supports the increased rate of fetal growth.

We want to make sure that you get all the notable nutrients of pregnancy. If you use our menus, you will get all of them you need, with the exception of iron (which we discussed above) and zinc at lower calorie levels. If you're planning your own meals, though, be sure to include those pregnancy superfoods you learned about in Chapter Four, which will help you meet these needs. For example, when you make a salad, take one more second to reach for the darkest green you can find. Spinach is always a superior choice green (rich in iron), for example, and romaine lettuce is good if you're not a spinach lover. Refer to the "About the Optimal Foods in the Optimal Pregnancy Diet" section of Chapter Four for foods that help you reel in all the nutrients. The other notable nutrients for this trimester that we would like to focus on particularly are protein and vitamin B_6, so necessary for the rapid tissue growth that is especially prominent as this trimester comes to a close.

EATING THE RIGHT NUMBER OF CALORIES

As you already learned, achieving just the right calorie intake during your pregnancy is key. That happy medium we keep mentioning is so critical! Trimester 2 is where the "pregnancy 300" comes in, when you especially need those extra 300 calories over your prepregnancy intake. That's why 2,200 calories is a good target for each day of this and your third trimester.

The 2,200-Calorie Level

We'd like you to start on this level because you're probably more active now, and your body and growing baby demand plenty of energy. If you find you're gaining more than 1 pound per week, cut back by 100-calorie increments, as we described in Chapter Four. Similarly, if you aren't gaining enough weight, then add in food by 100-calorie increments as we also explained in Chapter Four.

The 1,900-Calorie Level

If you find yourself just not particularly hungry on any given day, then we suggest following the lower 1,900-calorie menu. Don't just eliminate certain foods from the 2,200-calorie plan. Achieving the best calorie intake is important, but taking in all nutrients is equally critical. So you won't have to worry, we've planned more nutrient-dense foods at the lower calorie level. Also, if you are inactive or of very small stature, then the 1,900-calorie plan may be the better level for you. If you are gaining weight a little slowly at this level, add in extra calories in 100-calorie increments, as we explained in Chapter Four.

THE SECOND-TRIMESTER OPTIMAL DIET

As with the first-trimester chapter and the prepregnancy chapter, we've taken the guesswork out of getting all the nutrients you need. In this section, you'll find 2 weeks of daily meal plans specially designed to meet your needs in trimester 2. We've designed in the bigger breakfasts to satisfy your appetite as soon as you wake up, between-meal snacks to keep you from getting too hungry, and, best of all, a supertasty (and supernutritious) snack each day to keep those cravings at bay.

As you'll know if you used our meal plans in the earlier chapters, each breakfast in this trimester has the same calories as every other breakfast, and ditto for lunch and dinner. The breakfasts have 400 calories, the lunches have 500 calories, and the dinners have 550 calories. Therefore, you can mix up the breakfasts, lunches, and dinners within each calorie level so that you have enough different days' worth of menus to get you through the whole trimester. In fact, with 14 different choices for each breakfast, lunch, and dinner, you can make 2,744 different daily menus in each trimester! Refer back to the "How to Use Our Meal Plan" section on pages 92 through 93 for more information on using the meal plans. Note that all meal plan items in italics signify recipes that you'll find in Chapter Ten.

Day 1

	1,900 Calories	2,200 Calories
Breakfast	1 serving of *Cinnamon-Maple Brown Rice and Raisins*	
Morning Snack	2 fresh apricots (or 4 halves canned in juice)	
Lunch	*Lentil Salad*	
	1 cup skim milk	
Afternoon Snack	*Trail Mix III*	2 servings of *Trail Mix III* and 1½ cups skim milk
Dinner	1 serving of *Sweet and Sour Salmon Steaks*	
Evening Snack	*Chocolate Shake*	

Daily Nutrition Totals

Calories	1,897	2,223
Protein (g)	97	113
Carbohydrates (g)	293	346
Fiber (g)	37	43
Fat (g)	46	56
% calories from fat	21	22
Distribution of fat type:		
Saturated	15%	15%
Monounsaturated	65%	65%
Polyunsaturated	20%	20%
Vitamin B$_6$ (mg)	3.11	3.51
Folic acid (mcg)	705	783
Calcium (mg)	1,025	1,499
Iron (mg)	19	22
Zinc (mg)	10	13

g = gram(s); mcg = microgram(s); mg = milligram(s).

Day 2

	1,900 Calories	2,200 Calories
Breakfast	1 serving of *Creamed Eggs* ½ cup grapefruit juice	
Morning Snack	Tea Latte: 1 cup favorite decaf plain or flavored tea with 1 cup skim milk	
Lunch	*Sweet Walnut Wrap*	
	1 cup skim milk	
Afternoon Snack	1 banana	Peanut Butter–Banana Log: 2 tbsp. natural peanut butter and 2 tbsp. raisins on 1 banana
Dinner	3 oz. turkey breast	
	1 serving of *Herb and Apple Stuffing*	
	1 serving of *Cream Cheese Whipped Potatoes and Gravy*	
	8 steamed asparagus spears	
	1 cup skim milk	
Evening Snack	1 serving of *Orange Cream Fruit Tart*	

Daily Nutrition Totals		
Calories	1,956	2,218
Protein (g)	122	131
Carbohydrates (g)	292	315
Fiber (g)	30	34
Fat (g)	41	58
% calories from fat	18	23
Distribution of fat type:		
Saturated	25%	20%
Monounsaturated	38%	45%
Polyunsaturated	37%	35%
Vitamin B$_6$ (mg)	2.88	3.04
Folic acid (mcg)	632	683
Calcium (mg)	1,863	1,891
Iron (mg)	14	16
Zinc (mg)	11	12

g = gram(s); mcg = microgram(s); mg = milligram(s); oz. = ounce(s);
tbsp. = tablespoon(s).

Day 3

	1,900 Calories	2,200 Calories
Breakfast	1 serving of *Breakfast Strata*	
	1 cup skim milk	
	1 banana	
Morning Snack	1 serving of *Ready-to-go Fruit Salad*	
Lunch	Turkey Sandwich: 3 oz. turkey breast, 2 large romaine lettuce leaves, 2 tomato slices, 1 oz. low-fat cheese, and 2 tsp. honey mustard on 2 slices whole-wheat bread	
	1 cup fresh or frozen raspberries	
	1 cup skim milk	
Afternoon Snack	1 cup skim milk	¼ cup roasted sunflower seeds, 1½ cups skim milk
Dinner	Garden Cheeseburger: one 3-oz. Garden Burger patty, 1 oz. low-fat cheese, 1 cup watercress, 1 tomato slice, and 1 tsp. light mayonnaise on 1 hamburger bun	
	Chocolate Shake	
Evening Snack	*Frozen Lemonade*	

Daily Nutrition Totals		
Calories	1,966	2,185
Protein (g)	130	139
Carbohydrates (g)	324	336
Fiber (g)	36	39
Fat (g)	24	40
% calories from fat	10	16
Distribution of fat type:		
Saturated	40%	27%
Monounsaturated	30%	28%
Polyunsaturated	30%	47%
Vitamin B$_6$ (mg)	2.68	2.97
Folic acid (mcg)	484	565

Daily Nutrition Totals (continued)		
Calcium (mg)	2,475	2,615
Iron (mg)	14	15
Zinc (mg)	11	13

g = gram(s); mcg = microgram(s); mg = milligram(s); oz. = ounce(s);
tsp. = teaspoon(s).

Day 4

	1,900 Calories	*2,200 Calories*
Breakfast	*Craisin–Raisin Oatmeal*	
Morning Snack	*Peach Shake*	
Lunch	1 serving of *Raspberry Asparagus Quinoa Salad*	
	½ cup skim milk	
Afternoon Snack	*Veggie Salsa Snack*	
Dinner	1 serving of *The Best Hamburger*	
	½ cup skim milk	
Evening Snack	1 favorite flavor Newton cookie; 1 cup skim milk	1 serving of *Orange Cream Fruit Tart*

Daily Nutrition Totals		
Calories	1,959	2,215
Protein (g)	93	100
Carbohydrates (g)	298	330
Fiber (g)	29	29
Fat (g)	49	61
% calories from fat	22	24
Distribution of fat type:		
Saturated	28%	25%
Monounsaturated	56%	55%
Polyunsaturated	16%	20%
Vitamin B$_6$ (mg)	1.78	1.91
Folic acid (mcg)	545	588
Calcium (mg)	1,670	1,860

Iron (mg)	16	17
Zinc (mg)	12	13

g = gram(s); mcg = microgram(s); mg = milligram(s).

Day 5

	1,900 Calories	*2,200 Calories*
Breakfast	1 cup Total cereal with 2 tbsp. almonds, 1 cup blueberries, and 1 cup skim milk	
Morning Snack	1 papaya (approximately 11 oz. or 300 g)	1 papaya (approximately 11 oz. or 300 g), Tea Latte: 1 cup favorite decaf plain or flavored tea with 1 cup skim milk
Lunch	*Minted Strawberry Salad*	
	½ cup skim milk	
Afternoon Snack	2 graham crackers, 1½ cups skim milk	*Trail Mix III,* 1½ cups skim milk
Dinner	3 oz. grilled salmon	
	1 small baked potato with 2 tbsp. fat-free sour cream and 2 tbsp. chives	
	6 asparagus spears with 1 tsp. lemon juice	
	1 cup skim milk	
Evening Snack	1 serving of *Chocolate Fudge Brownies,* 1 cup skim milk	1 serving of *Chocolate Fudge Brownies,* 1½ cups skim milk

Daily Nutrition Totals		
Calories	1,900	2,183
Protein (g)	96	113
Carbohydrates (g)	285	343
Fiber (g)	45	55
Fat (g)	53	54
% calories from fat	24	21
Distribution of fat type:		
Saturated	19%	21%
Monounsaturated	62%	58%
Polyunsaturated	19%	21%

Daily Nutrition Totals (*continued*)		
Vitamin B$_6$ (mg)	4.73	5.14
Folic acid (mcg)	1,040	1,074
Calcium (mg)	2,171	2,752
Iron (mg)	33	36
Zinc (mg)	10	12

g = gram(s); mcg = microgram(s); mg = milligram(s); oz. = ounce(s);
tbsp. = tablespoon(s); tsp. = teaspoon(s).

Day 6		
	1,900 Calories	*2,200 Calories*
Breakfast	1 serving of *Ready-to-go Fruit Salad* with 1 cup extra-calcium low-fat cottage cheese	
	¾ cup calcium-fortified orange juice	
Morning Snack	1 slice whole-wheat toast with 1 tsp. favorite flavor jam or jelly	1 slice whole-wheat toast with 2 tsp. favorite flavor jam or jelly
Lunch	1 serving of *Arugula with Basil–Balsamic Dressing*	
	1½ cups skim milk	
	1 fresh peach (or 2 halves, canned in juice)	
Afternoon Snack	1 serving of *Orange–Spinach Salad*	1 serving of *Orange–Spinach Salad* sprinkled with ½ cup roasted pumpkin seeds
Dinner	One 4-oz. grilled pork chop	
	1 serving of *Cream Cheese Whipped Potatoes and Gravy*	
	1 cup steamed broccoli	
	1 cup skim milk	
	1 orange	
Evening Snack	Tea Latte: 1 cup favorite decaf plain or flavored tea with 1½ cups skim milk	2 chocolate chip cookies, 1½ cups skim milk

Daily Nutrition Totals		
Calories	1,936	2,232
Protein (g)	122	129
Carbohydrates (g)	293	333
Fiber (g)	40	43
Fat (g)	39	52
% calories from fat	17	20
Distribution of fat type:		
Saturated	27%	26%
Monounsaturated	40%	42%
Polyunsaturated	33%	32%
Vitamin B_6 (mg)	2.53	2.59
Folic acid (mcg)	684	701
Calcium (mg)	2,326	2,349
Iron (mg)	20	22
Zinc (mg)	10	13

g = gram(s); mcg = microgram(s); mg = milligram(s); oz. = ounce(s);
tsp. = teaspoon(s).

Day 7

	1,900 Calories	2,200 Calories
Breakfast	Egg–Cheese Breakfast Stack	
Morning Snack	½ cup Total cereal with ½ cup skim milk	1½ cups Total cereal with 1 cup skim milk and 1 tbsp. almonds
Lunch	1 serving of Cream of Broccoli Soup	
	1 small whole-wheat bagel	
	1 orange	
Afternoon Snack	1 cup pineapple chunks with ¼ cup fat-free vanilla yogurt	2 cups pineapple chunks with ¼ cup fat-free vanilla yogurt
Dinner	1 serving of Chicken Pasta Salad with Cilantro–Peanut Sauce	
	1 cup skim milk	
Evening Snack	Strawberry Milkshake	

Daily Nutrition Totals		
Calories	1,933	2,203
Protein (g)	128	138
Carbohydrates (g)	252	304
Fiber (g)	35	42
Fat (g)	53	57
% calories from fat	24	23
Distribution of fat type:		
Saturated	44%	21%
Monounsaturated	45%	47%
Polyunsaturated	11%	32%
Vitamin B_6 (mg)	3.28	5.82
Folic acid (mcg)	853	1,345
Calcium (mg)	2,318	2,778
Iron (mg)	24	46
Zinc (mg)	15	16

g = gram(s); mcg = microgram(s); mg = milligram(s); tbsp. = tablespoon(s).

Day 8		
	1,900 Calories	**2,200 Calories**
Breakfast	2 oat bran waffles with 1½ cups sliced strawberries and ¼ cup low-fat frozen whipped topping	
	1 cup skim milk	
Morning Snack	1 banana	*Trail Mix III*, ¾ cup calcium-fortified orange juice
Lunch	*Nutty Black Bean Salad*	
	1 cup skim milk	
Afternoon Snack	1 serving of *Strawberry Cheesecake*	1 serving of *Strawberry Cheesecake*, 1½ cups skim milk
Dinner	1 serving of *Classic Spaghetti*	
Evening Snack	1 orange	

Daily Nutrition Totals		
Calories	1,918	2,209
Protein (g)	109	122
Carbohydrates (g)	297	354
Fiber (g)	57	64
Fat (g)	42	44
% calories from fat	19	17
Distribution of fat type:		
Saturated	35%	35%
Monounsaturated	36%	36%
Polyunsaturated	29%	29%
Vitamin B$_6$ (mg)	2.73	2.52
Folic acid (mcg)	546	587
Calcium (mg)	1,402	2,083
Iron (mg)	21	25
Zinc (mg)	19	21

g = gram(s); mcg = microgram(s); mg = milligram(s).

Day 9

	1,900 Calories	*2,200 Calories*
Breakfast	1 small whole-wheat bagel with 1 tbsp. natural peanut butter	
	1 cup skim milk	
Morning Snack	1 papaya (approximately 11 oz. or 300 g)	
Lunch	*Guacamole Wrap*	
	1 cup skim milk	
Afternoon Snack	2 fresh apricots (or 4 halves canned in juice)	½ cup skim milk; Fruit Salad: 2 fresh apricots (or 4 halves canned in juice), 1 cup blueberries, ¼ cup fruit sorbet, and ¼ cup roasted sunflower seeds
Dinner	1 serving of *Roasted Chicken and Veggies*	
	½ cup skim milk	
Evening Snack	*Frozen Chocolate Banana Shake*	

Daily Nutrition Totals

Calories	1,901	2,257
Protein (g)	119	131
Carbohydrates (g)	303	348
Fiber (g)	46	53
Fat (g)	24	51
% calories from fat	15	19
Distribution of fat type:		
Saturated	21%	17%
Monounsaturated	58%	44%
Polyunsaturated	21%	39%
Vitamin B$_6$ (mg)	3.08	3.45
Folic acid (mcg)	493	596
Calcium (mg)	1,667	1,854
Iron (mg)	499	16
Zinc (mg)	13	15

g = gram(s); mcg = microgram(s); mg = milligram(s); oz. = ounce(s);
tbsp. = tablespoon(s).

Day 10

	1,900 Calories	**2,200 Calories**
Breakfast	*Mandarin Breakfast Broil*	
	1 cup skim milk	
Morning Snack	*Trail Mix III*	
Lunch	Peanut Butter Sandwich: 2 tbsp. natural peanut butter and 2 tsp. favorite jam or jelly on 2 slices whole-wheat bread	
	1 cup skim milk	
	2 kiwis	
Afternoon Snack	1 cup skim milk	1 favorite flavor Newton cookie; 1 cup skim milk
Dinner	1 serving of *Tuna Pasta*	
	6 whole-wheat crackers	

	1,900 Calories	*2,200 Calories*
Dinner (*cont.*)	1 cup skim milk	
	1 fresh peach	
Evening Snack	2 favorite flavor Newton cookies, decaf plain or flavored tea or coffee	*Banana Split*

Daily Nutrition Totals		
Calories	1,905	2,236
Protein (g)	109	114
Carbohydrates (g)	307	368
Fiber (g)	40	47
Fat (g)	35	45
% calories from fat	16	18
Distribution of fat type:		
Saturated	23%	31%
Monounsaturated	46%	44%
Polyunsaturated	31%	25%
Vitamin B$_6$ (mg)	1.75	2.57
Folic acid (mcg)	423	482
Calcium (mg)	1,911	2,046
Iron (mg)	17	18
Zinc (mg)	12	13

g = gram(s); mcg = microgram(s); mg = milligram(s); tbsp. = tablespoon(s); tsp. = teaspoon(s).

Day 11

	1,900 Calories	*2,200 Calories*
Breakfast	*Raspberry Banana Smoothie*	
	1 slice whole-wheat toast with 1 tsp. natural peanut butter	
Morning Snack	1 whole-wheat pita pocket with ¼ cup extra-calcium fat-free cottage cheese	1 whole-wheat pita pocket with ½ cup extra-calcium fat-free cottage cheese

Day 11 (continued)

	1,900 Calories	2,200 Calories
Lunch	Tomato Salad	
	1 serving of Chocolate Fudge Brownies	
	½ cup skim milk	
Afternoon Snack	2 tbsp. dry roasted peanuts	1 small baked potato with 1 tbsp. low-fat sour cream
Dinner	1 serving of Creamy Chicken Noodle Casserole	
	½ cup skim milk	
Evening Snack	1 cup sliced strawberries with 1 cup skim milk	2 tbsp. dry-roasted peanuts, 1 cup skim milk

Daily Nutrition Totals		
Calories	1,958	2,201
Protein (g)	111	121
Carbohydrates (g)	251	296
Fiber (g)	31	37
Fat (g)	64	66
% calories from fat	29	26
Distribution of fat type:		
Saturated	32%	33%
Monounsaturated	50%	48%
Polyunsaturated	18%	19%
Vitamin B$_6$ (mg)	2.39	2.91
Folic acid (mcg)	516	559
Calcium (mg)	1,478	1,654
Iron (mg)	16	18
Zinc (mg)	9	10

g = gram(s); mcg = microgram(s); mg = milligram(s); tbsp. = tablespoon(s); tsp. = teaspoon(s).

Day 12

	1,900 Calories	2,200 Calories
Breakfast	Apple Oatmeal	
	½ cup calcium-fortified orange juice	
Morning Snack	1 hard-boiled egg	
Lunch	1 serving of Spinach–Pear Salad	
	1 cup skim milk	
	2 Hershey's Kisses	
Afternoon Snack	1 cup Total cereal with 1 cup skim milk	1 cup Total cereal with ¼ cup raisins, ¼ cup roasted sunflower seeds, and 1 cup skim milk
Dinner	1 serving of Scalloped Potatoes	
	1 serving of Celery and Apple Salad	
Evening Snack	2 cups fresh or frozen raspberries with 1 tbsp. low-fat frozen whipped topping	

Daily Nutrition Totals		
Calories	1,916	2,226
Protein (g)	86	94
Carbohydrates (g)	309	350
Fiber (g)	49	55
Fat (g)	44	60
% calories from fat	20	23
Distribution of fat type:		
Saturated	24%	19%
Monounsaturated	41%	38%
Polyunsaturated	35%	43%
Vitamin B$_6$ (mg)	3.91	4.27
Folic acid (mcg)	870	947
Calcium (mg)	2,041	2,084
Iron (mg)	34	36
Zinc (mg)	13	15

g = gram(s); mcg = microgram(s); mg = milligram(s); tbsp. = tablespoon(s).

Day 13

	1,900 Calories	*2,200 Calories*
Breakfast	1 whole-wheat English muffin with ½ cup low-fat ricotta cheese swirled with 2 tsp. strawberry jam or jelly	
	½ pink grapefruit	
Morning Snack	1 orange	½ 6-oz. can tuna, canned in water, with 1 tsp. light mayonnaise and 1 tsp. relish on 4 whole-wheat crackers
Lunch	*Easy Cheesy Pasta Salad*	
	1 cup skim milk	
Afternoon Snack	¼ 6-oz. can tuna, canned in water, with 1 tsp. light mayonnaise and 1 tsp. relish on 3 whole-wheat crackers	1 serving of *Orange–Spinach Salad*
Dinner	4 oz. grilled salmon	
	1 serving of *Waldorf Salad*	
	1 small baked potato with 1 tsp. olive oil- or canola oil-based margarine	
Evening Snack	1 serving of *Orange–Spinach Salad*	*Strawberry Milkshake*

Daily Nutrition Totals		
Calories	1,953	2,215
Protein (g)	109	132
Carbohydrates (g)	226	265
Fiber (g)	34	39
Fat (g)	75	78
% calories from fat	33	31
Distribution of fat type:		
Saturated	35%	36%
Monounsaturated	36%	36%
Polyunsaturated	29%	28%
Vitamin B$_6$ (mg)	2.97	3.37
Folic acid (mcg)	868	907

Calcium (mg)	1,674	2,082
Iron (mg)	18	20
Zinc (mg)	11	13

g = gram(s); mcg = microgram(s); mg = milligram(s); oz. = ounce(s);
tsp. = teaspoon(s).

Day 14		
	1,900 Calories	*2,200 Calories*
Breakfast	¾ cup Fiber One cereal with 5 chopped dates, 2 tbsp. wheat germ, and 1 cup skim milk	
Morning Snack	1 banana	1 banana and 1 cup calcium-fortified orange juice
Lunch	*Chicken Wrap*	
	1 *Banana Chocolate Chip Muffin*	
Afternoon Snack	Tea Latte: 1 cup favorite decaf plain or flavored tea with 1 cup skim milk	2 oatmeal raisin cookies, 1½ cups skim milk
Dinner	1 serving of *Vegetarian Chili*	
	Salad of Many Greens (Side)	
	½ cup skim milk	
Evening Snack	*Peach Shake*	

Daily Nutrition Totals		
Calories	1,910	2,194
Protein (g)	105	110
Carbohydrates (g)	317	370
Fiber (g)	59	60
Fat (g)	40	45
% calories from fat	18	17
Distribution of fat type:		
Saturated	20%	20%
Monounsaturated	60%	60%
Polyunsaturated	20%	20%
Vitamin B$_6$ (mg)	3.65	3.84

Daily Nutrition Totals (continued)		
Folic acid (mcg)	654	713
Calcium (mg)	1,629	2,076
Iron (mg)	24	25
Zinc (mg)	13	14

g = gram(s); mcg = microgram(s); mg = milligram(s); tbsp. = tablespoon(s).

THE MEAL PLAN: DOING IT YOURSELF

You may want to use our meal plans every day of this trimester or you may want the freedom to plan your own meals occasionally or even every day. The first table below provides the number of servings from each food group, from dairy foods to fruits and vegetables, that you and your baby need each day. The table after contains our suggestions for dividing these servings up between meals and snacks for the day, to best satisfy your increased appetite. Of course, feel free to swap foods around according to your schedule and appetite. Please refer to Chapter Four, pages 94 through 96, for examples of serving sizes and to pages 93 through 94 for more advice on putting together your own meal plans.

Food Groups by Calorie Level

	1,900 Calories	*2,200 Calories*
Nonfat dairy	4 servings	5 servings
Whole-grain foods	6 servings	7 servings
Legumes	2 servings	3 servings
Fruits	3 servings	4 servings
Vegetable	5 servings	5 servings
Lean proteins	4 servings	4 servings
Nuts or seeds	2 oz. nuts or 4 oz. seeds	2 oz. nuts or 4 oz. seeds
Added fats	2 servings	3 servings

Food Groups by Meals

	1,900 Calories	*2,200 Calories*
Breakfast	2 whole grains 2 milks 1 lean protein 1 fruit	2 whole grains 2 milks 1 lean protein 2 fruits

	1,900 Calories	*2,200 Calories*
Morning Snack	1 milk	1 milk
	2 oz. nuts or 4 oz. seeds	2 oz. nuts or 4 oz. seeds
Lunch	2 whole grains	2 whole grains
	2 legumes	3 legumes
	3 vegetables	3 vegetables
		1 milk
Afternoon Snack	2 fruits	2 fruits
		1 whole grain
Dinner	2 whole grains	2 whole grains
	2 vegetables	2 vegetables
	3 lean proteins	3 lean proteins
Evening Snack	1 milk	1 milk
	2 fruits	2 fruits
As Desired	2 servings added fat	3 servings added fat

TROUBLESHOOTING

What Can I Do About Cravings?

There are cravings and then there are cravings. Some women desire tomatoes or celery, foods that will not have much of an impact on your calorie intake. Others have an unquenchable hankering for a piece of chocolate cake, but only occasionally; again, it won't do any harm if it is only every once in a while. But some pregnant women do develop frequent cravings for high-calorie, less nutritious foods. If this is you, we have a few tactics that may help you combat them.

First, be proactive about your cravings by using the strategies we've built into our meal plans: eating a filling breakfast everyday, avoiding hunger with between-meal snacks, and enjoying the treats we have planned in every day. Follow the time-honored rule of not shopping for groceries before a meal or when you're hungry. One more idea: Try a tall glass of water or large cup of decaf flavored tea to squelch an appetite.

If you just can't resist, think about lower-fat, lower-calorie ways to satisfy your craving. For example, if you must have ice cream, try stocking your freezer with fat-free frozen yogurt for a healthier treat. And if chocolate is your weakness, reach for a little Hershey's Kiss rather than a whole chocolate bar.

Iron Supplements Make Me Constipated; What Can I Do?

Adding extra fiber and water to your eating plan will help. Make sure you are drinking at least eight glasses of caffeine-free fluids daily. If you follow our menus, you should be getting enough fiber. If you are not, then try switching from white bread to whole grain, and also adding in more fruits and vegetables.

Iron Supplements Nauseate Me; What Can I Do?

Try taking your iron with a meal. You can also try taking it at night with your snack before bed, and then you will probably sleep through the nausea. Some women also find that it helps to divide up the iron into two or three smaller doses.

CHAPTER EIGHT

The Third-Trimester Optimal Diet

Anticipation for the birth of your child grows as you do. If you haven't already thought about names, perhaps you are now. You may be shopping for the nursery and constructing or redecorating a room.

The baby inside you has his or her final construction projects in progress, too. And that means he or she demands just the right number of calories, as well as notable nutrients, to complete them. Refer to the chapter sections "Mom's Changing Body" and "Baby's Construction Projects" for details on what is happening this trimester.

By this last third of your pregnancy, your stomach essentially competes with your baby for a limited amount of additional space in which to expand. In practical terms, this means it can be difficult to eat enough during this trimester because there is simply not enough room for your stomach. For this reason, you may also experience heartburn and other digestive problems; the "Troubleshooting" section at the end of this chapter discusses ways to minimize the discomfort they cause.

MOM'S CHANGING BODY

Month 7

In addition to symptoms previously experienced, you may have an itchy belly, increased breast tenderness, leg cramps, and numbness, tingling, or pain in your hands. You will probably still have a hearty appetite. Your moodiness will probably decrease, and you will become increasingly interested in learning about pregnancy, childbirth, and babies. As your baby's rate of growth picks up from this point forward, meeting your protein and nutrient needs becomes even more critical. As your baby grows, his or her blood supply must also increase, which means that getting the nutrients necessary to build healthy red blood cells comes to the fore as a goal.

Month 8

As your baby continues to grow, he or she will now push into the space where your lungs are, which can cause you to feel short of breath; the baby also moves into your stomach area, leading to that stuffed feeling we described earlier. As your hormones begin to change again and start to prepare you for delivery and nursing, you may have some colostrum leaking from your breasts and scattered Braxton Hicks contractions (when the uterus hardens for a period of about one minute before returning to normal). These hormonal changes can also cause hot flashes that are probably similar to those experienced during menopause. As your pregnancy progresses, you may experience difficulty sleeping because of heartburn, frequent urination, or not being able to get comfortable as your abdomen grows in girth. In some women, the weight of the baby can cause back and leg pain and may cause varicose veins to appear. You will continue to feel distinct fetal movement, and you can feel a range of emotions, from apprehension to excitement about your baby. Keeping up an adequate calorie and protein intake during these last stages of pregnancy is key to nourishing your baby properly. At the same time, you don't want to overeat. You may have a good appetite, in spite of the constant compression on your stomach, simply because baby is eating more, too. Be careful to stay within the calorie and weight gain recommendations we have provided for you in Chapter Three. Now and in the last month, getting plenty of folic acid is imperative, as this notable nutrient can help prevent premature delivery.

Month 9

You will feel strong and regular fetal activity in the ninth month of pregnancy. Your nesting instincts will increase, and you may enjoy spending more time shopping for baby items. It is normal to feel a mix of excitement about the approaching birth and anxiety over your baby's safety during delivery. You may experience increasingly heavy vaginal discharge, leaking urine, constipation, lower back pain, and more intense or frequent Braxton Hicks contractions. It can be difficult to sleep in your usual position for two reasons: your growing abdomen and also the shortness of breath. Sleeping slightly propped up on a couple of pillows can help alleviate your shortness of breath. Even though you may feel full to overflowing, it is still important to take in the optimal number of calories and grams of protein so that your baby can finish every last construction detail. In addition, taking in enough folic acid at this stage continues to be of the utmost importance to help prevent premature delivery.

BABY'S CONSTRUCTION PROJECTS

Month 7

At the seventh month, your baby will be about 13 inches long and weigh 1¾ pounds. The baby is covered with thin skin and has unique finger- and toeprints, and the eyelids are parted. His or her construction projects demand just the right number of calories, grams of protein, and other notable nutrients we mention below.

Month 8

At the eighth month of pregnancy, your baby weighs about 3 pounds. The baby can suck his or her thumb, hiccup, and cry and may respond to light, sound, and pain. At this point, the baby will be sufficiently developed to survive outside the womb with hospital support. Your baby gains weight rather rapidly now, so getting the right number of calories and grams of protein (and all the supporting nutrients) remains of critical importance.

Month 9

During the final month of your pregnancy, your baby will grow to be about 18 inches long and an average of 7.5 pounds. The baby's brain growth accelerates; he or she can see and hear, and most other systems are well developed. So although you will feel full on most days, you need to continue to feed your rapidly growing baby just the right amounts of calories and protein and nutrients to ensure that these construction projects are completed as perfectly as possible.

Nutrition Priorities

- Avoid under- and overnutrition; obtain an optimal number of calories
- Fill high protein needs
- Ensure adequate iron intake
- Focus again on folic acid
- Fill increasing calcium needs

Avoid Under- and Overnutrition; Obtain an Optimal Number of Calories

Avoiding both undernutrition and overnutrition gives the best chance that your baby will be born at an average weight, neither overly large nor overly small. For example, overnutrition in this trimester can cause your baby to be born heavier than the average; if your child is a girl, this can place her at increased risk for breast cancer. At the other end of the spectrum, undernutrition may lead to a smaller-than-average baby who may be at increased risk of heart disease or diabetes as an adult. The rate of weight gain to aim for in this trimester is around 1 pound per week—about 12 to 13 pounds for the trimester.

For most women, this is the only trimester that too many calories can be just as much of a problem as too few. Some days, you may still have a craving or two to satisfy, whereas on other days, you may just feel too full to eat. We hope we've provided you with enough ideas with which to get all the calories you need on those "I'm too full to eat" days, as well as strategies to appease those lingering cravings without overdoing it! For example, our menus emphasize eating between meals more than in any other trimester, meaning that the meals themselves are smaller and won't take up as much room in your stomach.

Fill High Protein Needs

Protein needs remain an absolute priority in the third trimester, as does the need for vitamin B_6, which your body requires to put that protein to good use. Your baby is gaining weight rapidly now, going from just a little over 1 pound at the beginning of this trimester to an average of 7.5 pounds at birth. This increase in weight doesn't just require calories: Your baby needs proteins to build healthy tissues, which will in turn build healthy organs. So in addition to getting enough calories, you need to take in enough protein to make sure that tissues form optimally. As we've said throughout this book, this also requires high amounts of several of the notable nutrients: vitamin B_6, zinc, and folic acid.

Ensure Adequate Iron Intake

During this trimester, your iron needs are the highest, and even though you might not have been anemic up to this point, you can still develop this common problem of pregnancy. Many women must start an iron supplement in the second trimester, but others don't need to until the final 3 months of pregnancy. Don't think you have a poor diet if you need an iron supplement; iron requirements are so high during pregnancy that it is almost impossible to meet them through diet alone. Do ask your obstetrician or nurse midwife about an appropriate iron supplement for you if you are anemic.

Focus Again on Folic Acid

Although getting enough folic acid throughout pregnancy is a nutritional priority, doing so in the last trimester—especially in the last month—is very important in preventing premature delivery. In studies, women who consumed fewer than 240 micrograms of folic acid daily were twice as likely to give birth prematurely as women consuming 240 micrograms or more.

If You Take Iron Supplements

If you become anemic and must take an iron supplement, ask your health-care provider about also taking zinc. Iron supplements of 60 milligrams may increase the need for zinc, because iron reduces your absorption of zinc. In turn, taking extra zinc bumps up your need for copper (for the same reason). Don't take more than 15 milligrams of zinc; 1.5 to 3.0 milligrams of copper is an optimal supplemental range.

Fill Increasing Calcium Needs

As your baby's bones form, he or she will draw the necessary calcium from your bones if you don't get enough of this nutrient every day. This leaves you at risk for osteoporosis later in life. By the way, even though yogurt and cheese are rich in calcium, we suggest you get much of your calcium from skim milk. This is because yogurt and cheese do not contain added vitamin D, which helps your body to absorb calcium. Why? Yogurt and cheese are made from milk before it is fortified with vitamin D.

THE THIRD-TRIMESTER OPTIMAL DIET

We've worked really hard to make sure you get all the nutrients you need during this third trimester and have designed 2 weeks of daily meal plans tailored to meet your needs when your baby is growing so rapidly but when you may feel you don't have enough room for all the food you need.

For instance, in this trimester, we've placed much of the bone-building but oh-so-filling milk between meals so that it doesn't interfere with your appetite. We've also moved many of the salads—one of the best sources of the notable nutrient folic acid—between meals, also so that you aren't so full at mealtime. In addition, you'll find more nuts and seeds than in the previous chapters; they are both nutrient- and calorie-dense foods that help meet nutrient and energy needs without making you feel so full.

As you'll know if you used our meal plans in the other chapters, each breakfast is interchangeable with every other breakfast, and each lunch with the other lunches; ditto for the dinners. Pardon us if you've read this before, but we feel this is important, so we're going to repeat it just in case you are starting with our meal plans this trimester. This allows you to mix up the breakfasts, lunches, and dinners within each calorie level so that you have enough different days' worth of menus to get you through the whole trimester. Here's a breakdown of total calories in each of the meals regardless of calorie level:

- Breakfast: 400 calories
- Lunch: 500 calories
- Dinner: 550 calories

More information on using our meal plans can be found on pages 92 through 93. Note that all meal plan items in italics signify recipes that you'll find in Chapter Ten.

Day 1

	1,900 Calories	*2,200 Calories*
Breakfast	1 serving of *Individual Pumpkin Pie Custards* sprinkled with 2 tbsp. almonds	
	½ cup skim milk	
Morning Snack	Tea Latte: 1 cup decaf plain or flavored tea with 1 cup skim milk	*Peach Shake*
Lunch	1 serving of *Taste of Summer Vegetable Lentil Soup*	
	1½ cups skim milk	
	2 fresh apricots (or 4 halves canned in juice)	
Afternoon Snack	1 serving of *Celery and Apple Salad*	1 serving of *Celery and Apple Salad* with 3 tbsp. roasted sunflower seeds
Dinner	1 serving of *Chicken Pot Pie Without the Pie*	
Evening Snack	1 serving of *Strawberry Cheesecake*	

Daily Nutrition Totals		
Calories	1,943	2,221
Protein (g)	118	126
Carbohydrates (g)	290	329
Fiber (g)	42	47
Fat (g)	42	54
% calories from fat	19	21
Distribution of fat type:		
Saturated	22%	20%
Monounsaturated	56%	45%
Polyunsaturated	22%	35%
Vitamin B$_6$ (mg)	2.7	2.84
Folic acid (mcg)	486	538
Calcium (mg)	1,785	1,860
Iron (mg)	17	18
Zinc (mg)	11	12

g = gram(s); mcg = microgram(s); mg = milligram(s); tbsp. = tablespoon(s).

Day 2

	1,900 Calories	**2,200 Calories**
Breakfast	Raspberry Banana Smoothie	
Morning Snack	1 serving of *Ready-to-go Fruit Salad*	1 serving of *Ready-to-go Fruit Salad,* 3 favorite flavor Newton cookies
Lunch	Carrot–Tuna Pita	
	1 cup skim milk	
Afternoon Snack	1 serving of *Rainbow Side Salad*	
Dinner	Peanut Papaya Pasta Salad	
Evening Snack	1 favorite flavor Newton cookie, 1½ cups skim milk	*Peanut Butter– Chocolate Shake*

Daily Nutrition Totals		
Calories	1,884	2,236
Protein (g)	109	123
Carbohydrates (g)	272	296
Fiber (g)	47	51
Fat (g)	47	70
% calories from fat	22	27
Distribution of fat type:		
Saturated	15%	17%
Monounsaturated	60%	58%
Polyunsaturated	25%	25%
Vitamin B$_6$ (mg)	3.25	3.23
Folic acid (mcg)	581	649
Calcium (mg)	1,665	1,461
Iron (mg)	19	20
Zinc (mg)	11	11

g = gram(s); mcg = microgram(s); mg = milligram(s).

Day 3

	1,900 Calories	*2,200 Calories*
Breakfast	1 serving of *Strawberry Cheesecake*	
	½ cup calcium-fortified orange juice	
Morning Snack	½ cup Total cereal with 1 banana and ¾ cup skim milk	
Lunch	*Stuffed Peppers*	
	1 cup skim milk	
	1 kiwi	
Afternoon Snack	1 serving of *Simple Garden Salad*	1 serving of *Simple Garden Salad* with ⅓ cup roasted sunflower seeds
Dinner	4 oz. grilled salmon	
	1 serving of *Herbed Garlic Cheese Bread*	
Evening Snack	*Creamy Orange Shake*	1 serving of *Orange Cream Fruit Tart*

Daily Nutrition Totals

Calories	1,929	2,250
Protein (g)	101	104
Carbohydrates (g)	292	299
Fiber (g)	28	33
Fat (g)	42	76
% calories from fat	19	30
Distribution of fat type:		
Saturated	29%	21%
Monounsaturated	47%	40%
Polyunsaturated	24%	39%
Vitamin B$_6$ (mg)	3.62	3.84
Folic acid (mcg)	768	784
Calcium (mg)	1,694	1,470
Iron (mg)	22	25
Zinc (mg)	13	14

g = gram(s); mcg = microgram(s); mg = milligram(s); oz. = ounce(s).

Day 4

	1,900 Calories	*2,200 Calories*
Breakfast	1 cup Raisin Bran cereal with 1 tbsp. chopped walnuts and 1 cup skim milk	
Morning Snack	1 papaya (about 11 oz. or 300 g)	1 papaya (about 11 oz. or 300 g), 1 cup skim milk
Lunch	1 serving of *Spinach–Pear Salad*	
	1 cup skim milk	
	1 fresh peach	
Afternoon Snack	4 dried Brazil nuts	*Veggie Salsa Snack,* 4 dried Brazil nuts
Dinner	3 oz. roast beef	
	1 serving of *Sweet-Potato Fries*	
	1 cup steamed broccoli	
Evening Snack	*Peanut Butter–Chocolate Shake*	

Daily Nutrition Totals

Calories	1,926	2,221
Protein (g)	97	112
Carbohydrates (g)	240	283
Fiber (g)	38	43
Fat (g)	74	82
% calories from fat	33	32
Distribution of fat type:		
Saturated	17%	18%
Monounsaturated	48%	46%
Polyunsaturated	35%	36%
Vitamin B$_6$ (mg)	2.48	3.02
Folic acid (mcg)	639	750
Calcium (mg)	1,213	1,675
Iron (mg)	21	23
Zinc (mg)	16	17

g = gram(s); mcg = microgram(s); mg = milligram(s); oz. = ounce(s); tbsp. = tablespoon(s).

Day 5

	1,900 Calories	2,200 Calories
Breakfast	2 poached eggs	
	2 slices whole-wheat toast with 2 tsp. olive oil- or canola oil-based margarine	
	1 pink grapefruit	
Morning Snack	Tea Latte: 1 cup decaf plain or flavored tea with 1 cup skim milk	2 oz. oat bran pretzels, 1½ cups skim milk
Lunch	1 serving of *Quinoa Roasted Red Pepper Salad*	
	1 cup skim milk	
Afternoon Snack	1 serving of *Ready-to-go Fruit Salad*	
Dinner	4 oz. skinless chicken breast	
	1 serving of *Cream Cheese Whipped Potatoes and Gravy*	
	8 asparagus spears	
	1 cup skim milk	
	1 orange	
Evening Snack	1 serving of *Strawberry Cheesecake*	

Daily Nutrition Totals		
Calories	1,971	2,231
Protein (g)	119	128
Carbohydrates (g)	283	331
Fiber (g)	29	33
Fat (g)	46	50
% calories from fat	21	20
Distribution of fat type:		
Saturated	32%	29%
Monounsaturated	42%	47%
Polyunsaturated	21%	24%
Vitamin B$_6$ (mg)	2.54	2.58
Folic acid (mcg)	544	549
Calcium (mg)	1,640	1,757
Iron (mg)	18	19
Zinc (mg)	12	12

g = gram(s); mcg = microgram(s); mg = milligram(s); oz. = ounce(s); tsp. = teaspoon(s).

Day 6

	1,900 Calories	*2,200 Calories*
Breakfast	1 serving of *Breakfast Strata*	
	1½ cups skim milk	
	2 kiwis	
Morning Snack	¼ cup almonds	¾ cup bran flakes cereal with ¼ cup almonds and 1 cup skim milk
Lunch	*Hummus Wrap*	
	1 cup skim milk	
Afternoon Snack	½ cup bran flakes cereal with ½ cup skim milk	1 serving of *Celery and Apple Salad*
Dinner	1 serving of *Tuna Melt*	
	1 serving of *Rainbow Side Salad*	
	½ cup skim milk	
Evening Snack	1 serving of *Orange Cream Fruit Tart*	

Daily Nutrition Totals		
Calories	1,925	2,215
Protein (g)	109	117
Carbohydrates (g)	253	321
Fiber (g)	44	51
Fat (g)	65	66
% calories from fat	29	25
Distribution of fat type:		
Saturated	20%	20%
Monounsaturated	56%	55%
Polyunsaturated	24%	25%
Vitamin B$_6$ (mg)	2.71	3.08
Folic acid (mcg)	671	748
Calcium (mg)	1,860	2,113
Iron (mg)	30	38
Zinc (mg)	16	18

g = gram(s); mcg = microgram(s); mg = milligram(s).

Day 7

	1,900 Calories	2,200 Calories
Breakfast	Apple Oatmeal	
	½ cup calcium-fortified orange juice	
Morning Snack	1 banana	Fruit Salad: 1 sliced banana with 1 cup sliced strawberries
Lunch	Tomato Salad	
	Vanilla Apricot Smoothie	
Afternoon Snack	1 small whole-wheat bagel with 1 tsp. natural peanut butter, 1½ cups skim milk	
Dinner	1 serving of The Best Hamburger	
Evening Snack	Strawberry–Spinach Salad: 2 cups chopped fresh spinach (or bagged fresh baby spinach) with 2 cups sliced strawberries and drizzled with 2 tbsp. calcium-fortified orange juice	1 serving of Orange–Spinach Salad sprinkled with 2 tbsp. roasted sunflower seeds

Daily Nutrition Totals

Calories	1,952	2,203
Protein (g)	87	97
Carbohydrates (g)	265	269
Fiber (g)	37	40
Fat (g)	67	92
% calories from fat	30	36
Distribution of fat type:		
Saturated	31%	25%
Monounsaturated	54%	50%
Polyunsaturated	15%	25%
Vitamin B$_6$ (mg)	2.3	2.76
Folic acid (mcg)	562	913
Calcium (mg)	1,720	1,857
Iron (mg)	17	22
Zinc (mg)	13	15

g = gram(s); mcg = microgram(s); mg = milligram(s); tbsp. = tablespoon(s); tsp. = teaspoon(s).

Day 8

	1,900 Calories	**2,200 Calories**
Breakfast	*Cheesy Mushroom Omelet*	
	2 slices whole-wheat toast with 1 tsp. olive oil– or canola oil–based margarine	
	1 cup skim milk	
Morning Snack	1 papaya (about 11 oz. or 300 g)	
Lunch	*Power Yogurt*	
	3 crispbread crackers	
Afternoon Snack	⅓ cup roasted sunflower seeds	⅓ cup roasted sunflower seeds, 4 crispbread crackers
Dinner	One 4-oz. grilled tuna steak	
	1 serving of *Sweet Potatoes in an Orange–Brown Sugar Glaze*	
	1 cup steamed green beans with 1 tbsp. almonds	
Evening Snack	½ cup Multi-Grain Cheerios with ½ cup skim milk	*Strawberry Milkshake*

Daily Nutrition Totals

Calories	1,909	2,186
Protein (g)	105	117
Carbohydrates (g)	273	332
Fiber (g)	38	48
Fat (g)	50	52
% calories from fat	23	21
Distribution of fat type:		
Saturated	14%	17%
Monounsaturated	41%	39%
Polyunsaturated	45%	44%
Vitamin B$_6$ (mg)	2.92	3.04
Folic acid (mcg)	462	497
Calcium (mg)	1,333	1,626
Iron (mg)	16	15
Zinc (mg)	12	13

g = gram(s); mcg = microgram(s); mg = milligram(s); oz. = ounce(s);
tbsp. = tablespoon(s); tsp. = teaspoon(s).

Day 9

	1,900 Calories	2,200 Calories
Breakfast	1 small whole-wheat bagel with 1 tbsp. natural peanut butter and 2 tsp. jam or jelly	
	1½ cups skim milk	
Morning Snack	1 banana	1 banana, 2 tbsp. almonds
Lunch	Carrot–Tuna Pita	
	1½ cups skim milk	
Afternoon Snack	1 serving of *Rainbow Side Salad*	2 cups sliced strawberries with 1 sliced kiwi
Dinner	1 serving of *Cheesy Spinach Pizza*	
Evening Snack	2 cups sliced strawberries with 1 sliced kiwi, 1 cup skim milk	*Peach Shake*

Daily Nutrition Totals		
Calories	1,976	2,216
Protein (g)	105	111
Carbohydrates (g)	298	336
Fiber (g)	43	48
Fat (g)	50	58
% calories from fat	22	23
Distribution of fat type:		
Saturated	30%	27%
Monounsaturated	45%	50%
Polyunsaturated	25%	23%
Vitamin B$_6$ (mg)	3.17	3.13
Folic acid (mcg)	760	766
Calcium (mg)	1,719	1,826
Iron (mg)	20	21
Zinc (mg)	12	12

g = gram(s); mcg = microgram(s); mg = milligram(s); tbsp. = tablespoon(s); tsp. = teaspoon(s).

Day 10

	1,900 Calories	**2,200 Calories**
Breakfast	½ cup extra calcium low-fat cottage cheese with 1 cup sliced strawberries	
	1 whole-wheat English muffin with 2 tsp. margarine	
	1 cup skim milk	
Morning Snack	1 serving of *Ready-to-go Fruit Salad*	
Lunch	*Rice and Asparagus Salad*	
Afternoon Snack	½ cup corn flakes cereal with ½ cup skim milk	*Trail Mix I*, ¾ cup corn flakes with 1 cup skim milk
Dinner	1 serving of *Roasted Chicken and Veggies*	
	½ cup skim milk	
Evening Snack	1 serving of *Orange–Spinach Salad*	

Daily Nutrition Totals

Calories	1,936	2,212
Protein (g)	108	118
Carbohydrates (g)	273	322
Fiber (g)	44	47
Fat (g)	54	60
% calories from fat	24	23
Distribution of fat type:		
Saturated	19%	21%
Monounsaturated	45%	44%
Polyunsaturated	36%	35%
Vitamin B$_6$ (mg)	3.42	3.67
Folic acid (mcg)	994	1,047
Calcium (mg)	1,518	1,697
Iron (mg)	20	21
Zinc (mg)	11	12

g = gram(s); mcg = microgram(s); mg = milligram(s); tsp. = teaspoon(s).

Day 11

	1,900 Calories	2,200 Calories
Breakfast	1 cup Total cereal with 1 sliced banana, 2 tbsp. chopped walnuts, and 1 cup skim milk	
Morning Snack	3 fresh apricots (or 6 halves canned in juice)	
Lunch	1 serving of *Orange–Spinach Salad*	
	1½ cups skim milk	
Afternoon Snack	*Karin's Banana Breakfast Frappé*	
Dinner	1 serving of *Roasted Red Pepper and Beef Wraps*	
	1 serving of *Rainbow Side Salad*	
Evening Snack	1 serving of *Individual Pumpkin Pie Custards*	2 servings of *Individual Pumpkin Pie Custards* sprinkled with 2 tbsp. chopped walnuts

Daily Nutrition Totals

Calories	1,950	2,220
Protein (g)	116	127
Carbohydrates (g)	279	318
Fiber (g)	33	35
Fat (g)	51	61
% calories from fat	23	23
Distribution of fat type:		
Saturated	21%	19%
Monounsaturated	51%	47%
Polyunsaturated	28%	34%
Vitamin B$_6$ (mg)	5.72	5.88
Folic acid (mcg)	927	951
Calcium (mg)	2,159	2,352
Iron (mg)	36	38
Zinc (mg)	14	16

g = gram(s); mcg = microgram(s); mg = milligram(s); tbsp. = tablespoon(s).

Day 12

	1,900 Calories	*2,200 Calories*
Breakfast	1 serving of *Individual Pumpkin Pie Custards* sprinkled with 1 tbsp. almonds	
Morning Snack	1 papaya (about 11 oz. or 300 g)	1 cup Total cereal with ½ cup roasted pumpkin seeds and 1 cup skim milk
Lunch	*Guacamole Wrap*	
	1 cup skim milk	
Afternoon Snack	1 cup Total cereal with 1 cup skim milk	*Veggie Salsa Snack*
Dinner	*Fresh 'n' Fruity Chicken Pasta*	
	1 cup skim milk	
Evening Snack	½ cup roasted pumpkin seeds	*Vanilla Apricot Smoothie*

Daily Nutrition Totals

Calories	1,976	2,199
Protein (g)	85	106
Carbohydrates (g)	326	354
Fiber (g)	39	42
Fat (g)	44	47
% calories from fat	20	19
Distribution of fat type:		
Saturated	22%	24%
Monounsaturated	39%	31%
Polyunsaturated	39%	35%
Vitamin B$_6$ (mg)	3.77	4.22
Folic acid (mcg)	900	903
Calcium (mg)	2,031	2,399
Iron (mg)	33	37
Zinc (mg)	13	14

g = gram(s); mcg = microgram(s); mg = milligram(s); oz. = ounce(s); tbsp. = tablespoon(s).

Day 13

	1,900 Calories	*2,200 Calories*
Breakfast	*Craisin–Raisin Oatmeal*	
Morning Snack	1 banana	
Lunch	*Peanut Papaya Pasta Salad*	
Afternoon Snack	Café Latte: 1 cup decaf coffee with 1 cup skim milk	½ cup bran flakes cereal with 1 cup skim milk and ¼ cup sunflower seeds
Dinner	1 serving of *Roasted Red Pepper and Trout Roll-Ups*	
Evening Snack	1 serving of *Orange–Spinach Salad*	

Daily Nutrition Totals		
Calories	1,973	2,223
Protein (g)	111	119
Carbohydrates (g)	252	275
Fiber (g)	35	41
Fat (g)	62	78
% calories from fat	28	31
Distribution of fat type:		
Saturated	19%	17%
Monounsaturated	50%	44%
Polyunsaturated	30%	39%
Vitamin B$_6$ (mg)	2.75	3.36
Folic acid (mcg)	818	963
Calcium (mg)	1,241	1,273
Iron (mg)	16	30
Zinc (mg)	10	14

g = gram(s); mcg = microgram(s); mg = milligram(s).

Day 14

	1,900 Calories	2,200 Calories
Breakfast	1 cup Fiber One cereal with 1 cup fresh or frozen raspberries, 1 tbsp. almonds, and 1 cup skim milk	
Morning Snack	1 orange	1 orange, ¼ cup dry-roasted peanuts
Lunch	Ham and Cheese Sandwich: 3 oz. lean ham, 1 oz. low-fat Swiss cheese, 2 large romaine lettuce leaves, and 2 tomato slices on 2 slices whole-wheat bread	
	1 cup skim milk	
	1 cup grapes	
Afternoon Snack	2 favorite flavor Newton cookies, ½ cup skim milk	2 favorite flavor Newton cookies, 1 cup skim milk
Dinner	1 serving of *Lentil Vegetable Stew*	
	Salad of Many Greens (Side)	
Evening Snack	*Chocolate Shake*	

Daily Nutrition Totals		
Calories	1,942	2,198
Protein (g)	91	104
Carbohydrates (g)	334	347
Fiber (g)	71	74
Fat (g)	39	60
% calories from fat	17	22
Distribution of fat type:		
Saturated	22%	21%
Monounsaturated	64%	58%
Polyunsaturated	14%	21%
Vitamin B$_6$ (mg)	2.53	2.68
Folic acid (mcg)	662	721
Calcium (mg)	1,784	1,954
Iron (mg)	24	25
Zinc (mg)	11	12

g = gram(s); mcg = microgram(s); mg = milligram(s); oz. = ounce(s); tbsp. = tablespoon(s).

THE MEAL PLAN: DOING IT YOURSELF

As with every other trimester, you have the option of using our meal plans every day or planning your own meals, whether just on the occasional day or throughout the trimester. Here, we give you the tools you need to plan meals without using our suggested menus.

The table "Food Groups by Calorie Level" provides the number of servings from each food group, from dairy foods and whole-grain foods to legumes and lean protein. Planning meals with these numbers of servings in mind will allow you to meet all your (and your baby's) nutrition requirements. The table after it is our suggestion for dividing these servings up between meals and snacks for the day, to best help you get in all your nutrition without ever feeling terribly full. Refer to Chapter Four, pages 94 through 96, to find information on serving sizes, and to pages 93 through 94, for advice on creating your own meal plans.

Food Groups by Calorie Level

	1,900 Calories	*2,200 Calories*
Nonfat dairy	4 servings	5 servings
Whole-grain foods	5 servings	6 servings
Legumes	2 servings	3 servings
Fruits	3 servings	4 servings
Vegetable	4 servings	4 servings
Lean proteins	4 servings	4 servings
Nuts or seeds	3 oz. nuts or 6 oz. seeds	3 oz. nuts or 6 oz. seeds
Added fats	2 tsp.	3 tsp.

oz. = ounce(s); tsp. = teaspoon(s).

Food Groups by Meals

	1,900 Calories	*2,200 Calories*
Breakfast	2 whole grains 1 lean protein 1 fruit	2 whole grains 1 lean protein 1 fruit
Morning Snack	1½ milk 2 fruits	1½ milk 2 fruits
Lunch	2 whole grains 2 legumes 1 vegetable	2 whole grains 3 legumes 1 vegetable ½ milk

(continued)

Food Groups by Meals (continued)

	1,900 Calories	2,200 Calories
Afternoon Snack	1 milk	1½ milk
	2 vegetables (as salad)	2 vegetables (as salad)
	3 oz. nuts or	3 oz. nuts or
	6 oz. seeds (for salad)	6 oz. seeds (for salad)
Dinner	1 whole grain	2 whole grains
	1 vegetable	1 vegetable
	3 lean proteins	3 lean proteins
Evening Snack	1½ milk	1½ milk
		1 fruit
As Desired	2 tsp. added fats	3 tsp. added fats

oz. = ounce(s); tsp. = teaspoon(s).

TROUBLESHOOTING

But There's No Room!

We totally understand the no-room-to-eat excuse for not eating, so we've devised menus that take this problem into account.

At first glance, our menus may seem a little odd. You'll find salads and milk between meals, and we've used a few more nut and seed servings than in the previous trimesters. It is by these strategies that we managed to work in enough calories each day—without causing you to feel too full at any one time. But we left regular evening meals in this plan so you can still cook the same meal for you and your partner, or your entire family, even though you will naturally want to eat less than a full meal at this time. You may also see a few more shakes and smoothies on the menu; this is another way of providing you with nutrient-packed calories.

One more word to the wise: Move your meals and snacks around as you need to. In particular, liquids, including bone-building milk, can fill you up in a big hurry. Spread these liquids out even further if you need to, leaving more room for the nutrient-rich foods you and your baby crave at this time.

I Seem to Have Perpetual Heartburn—Help!

Heartburn is caused by the same space issue that makes you feel full all the time: The baby's growing body can push on the contents of your stomach so much that they overpower the valve (called the sphincter) that generally keeps food from traveling backward up into the esophagus, or the tube that carries food from the mouth to the stomach. Unfortunately, by the time food backs up from the stomach into the esophagus, it is already mixed with stomach acid. This is why you feel a burning sensation, also called heartburn.

To ease your discomfort, you might want to divide your food into six smaller meals rather than three meals and three snacks. You can take some food from breakfast and move it to the morning snack, some from lunch and move it to the afternoon snack, and some from dinner to have with your evening snack. Some women find it helpful to avoid pepper and other foods that seem to increase heartburn. Also, even decaf coffee and tea can contribute to your heartburn, so you might try eliminating them if you are still faced with bothersome heartburn. One last piece of advice: Try to avoid drinking liquids at mealtimes. This means your stomach will be less full, reducing the chance of heartburn.

My Heartburn Seems to Be Worse When I Lie Down in Bed; Any Suggestions?

Sometimes, raising up the head of the bed with equal-size books (such as two phone books) under the two legs at the head end will place you at enough of an incline to help reduce heartburn. Just make sure they are secure so that the bed doesn't slip. This seems to work better than propping yourself up on pillows. One other thing: try to have your evening snack at least 1 or 2 hours before bed, so that your food has a chance to digest before you lie down.

I'm Eating Fiber-Rich Foods but Am Still Constipated; What Can I Do?

You're not alone if you have this problem. As the baby grows, he or she sits on your intestinal tract and rectum. As you can imagine, this can be incredibly constipating. We've worked in plenty of fiber into our meal plans, but even this may not be enough to solve the problem. If you are eating at least 25 grams of fiber every day (look at the nutrition information at the bottom of each meal plan) and drinking plenty of liquids, then ask your obstetrician or nurse midwife for another solution. Although many laxatives can be safe, others are not, so you should take one only on your health care provider's advice.

CHAPTER NINE

Special Guidelines for Women with Diabetes or Gestational Diabetes

Diabetes mellitus, a condition in which the body cannot regulate blood sugar (glucose) levels, is problematic for anyone affected. But abnormal blood sugar levels are even more of a problem for pregnant women. I'd like to explain gestational diabetes (the name for diabetes when it occurs for the first time during pregnancy), why it can occur in a woman who never had a hint of blood sugar abnormalities before pregnancy, the problems gestational diabetes can cause in a mom and her baby, when and how you should be checked for gestational diabetes, and the main management strategies.

Before I continue, I want to give you some critically important advice—so important that I will repeat it several times throughout this chapter. Make sure you are tested for gestational diabetes at the appropriate time in your pregnancy (generally between the twenty-fourth and twenty-eighth week of pregnancy). If you have gestational diabetes, you *must* seek the individualized medical *and* nutritional care you need to manage your diet and to check on your baby's health. No, I do not want to frighten you, but I do want to make sure that you don't simply take the information from this chapter as the sole advice for dealing with this condition.

Yes, this information is serious, and I don't want to take away from your joy of bringing a new life into this world, but you need to know these details. Knowing about the disease and how to manage it can help you have a healthy baby, even if you do develop gestational diabetes.

And one more important detail: If you have type 1 diabetes (insulin-dependent diabetes mellitus), you require specialized care that is beyond the scope of this book. Your diabetes specialist and obstetrician can coordinate the care you need.

Diabetes Basics

What follows below are just a few facts about blood sugar and diabetes. Please refer back to Chapter Two for greater detail.

- Everyone must always have some sugar, or glucose, in the bloodstream. Normal levels are between 60 and 120 milligrams per deciliter. We need sugar in the bloodstream so that our brains maintain clear thinking and that our body has enough energy, or fuel, to move and even to sit.
- One hundred percent of all the carbohydrates we eat, from rice to bananas to whole-grain bagels, is converted to blood glucose, just at different rates.
- Fifty-eight percent of the protein we eat is eventually, over a couple of hours, converted to blood glucose.
- Just 10% of the fat we eat is converted to blood glucose.
- The body produces a hormone called insulin to move the glucose from inside the bloodstream into the cells, where it can be used. Think of the insulin as the key that turns food into energy.
- Normally, the body has an incredible ability to regulate blood sugar levels. When the body's glucose "radar screen" senses more blood sugar in the bloodstream than is normal, the pancreas pumps out the requisite amounts of insulin to shuttle sugar from the blood into the cells and to therefore keep blood sugar levels in the normal ranges.
- If the pancreas does not produce enough insulin and blood sugar cannot be moved out of the bloodstream (which happens in diabetes), then two major things occur: The body does not get the energy it needs, and blood sugars remain higher than normal.
- The body gets rid of excess sugar in the bloodstream by filtering it out through the kidneys and into the urine, which passes from the body. The problem with this? It places considerable wear and tear on the kidneys, as well as on all the organs in the body.

GESTATIONAL DIABETES: AN EXPLANATION

Gestational diabetes occurs in approximately 3% to 5% of pregnant women in the United States, according to the latest statistics from the National Institutes of Health.

Three Types of Diabetes

Just to make a complicated topic even more confusing, there are three distinct types of diabetes mellitus. They are

- *Juvenile-onset, or insulin-dependent, diabetes mellitus:* This type of diabetes, also called type 1 diabetes, generally starts during childhood or adolescence because the pancreas stops producing insulin. All people with type 1 diabetes need insulin by injection or by pump and they have to follow individualized dietary guidelines. About 10% of all people who have diabetes have type 1 diabetes.
- *Adult-onset, or non-insulin-dependent, diabetes mellitus, (also called type 2 diabetes):* This type of diabetes generally occurs after age 40, commonly in people who are overweight, and/ or have a family history of diabetes. Type 2 diabetes can be managed with dietary modifications, dietary modifications with oral medications, or dietary modifications with injected insulin. Often, losing excess weight will greatly improve blood sugars and eliminate the need for medication or insulin. Somewhat confusingly, adult-onset diabetes is termed non-insulin-dependent diabetes even though some people who have it need insulin.
- *Gestational diabetes:* This is diabetes that begins for the first time during pregnancy in a woman who did not have blood sugar abnormalities before becoming pregnant.

As you learned in Chapter Two, and as we explained briefly above, the hormone insulin is a key player in regulating blood sugar levels. In pregnancy—in all women—insulin works at an advantage. Let me explain.

The placenta, that wonderful cocoon that nourishes your baby, produces a host of hormones that are vital to you and baby during pregnancy. Although absolutely necessary, some of these hormones inhibit the effect of insulin. In particular, estrogen, cortisol, and human placental lactogen block the insulin. In medical language, we say that these hormones have a contrainsular (against insulin) effect.

Most of the time, this contrainsular effect does not occur until about

Diabetes Complications

Although diabetes occurs silently—often causing no symptoms—sugar-rich blood coursing through the body causes a host of complications, including

- *Blindness or other eye complications:* Diabetes is the leading cause of new cases of blindness in people between the ages of 20 and 74.
- *Kidney damage:* Diabetes is the leading cause of serious kidney disease, accounting for about 40% of the nearly 28,000 people newly diagnosed in the United States yearly.
- *Nerve damage and amputations:* A person with diabetes is 15 to 40 times more likely to have an amputation of a toe, foot, or leg than is someone without diabetes. Each year, 56,000 people with diabetes have such an amputation.
- *Heart disease or stroke:* People with diabetes are two to four times more likely to have atherosclerotic heart disease. Stroke risk is also doubled to quadrupled.

midway through the pregnancy, at about 20 to 24 weeks. As you have learned in this book, the placenta grows throughout your pregnancy, expanding to meet your growing baby's needs. At around 20 to 24 weeks of gestation, the placenta makes a quantity of hormones that can significantly overpower the action of insulin. Medical experts refer to this as insulin resistance.

Why do some women get gestational diabetes but others do not? In most women, the pancreas simply pumps out increased amounts of insulin to keep blood sugars in check. Some pregnant women, however, cannot meet the demand. When the pancreas makes all the insulin it can and there still isn't enough to overcome the effect of the placenta's hormones, gestational diabetes results. After pregnancy, when the hormones of pregnancy no longer surge through a woman's body, insulin works as it used to, and the diabetes generally disappears. (Do note, however, that women who have experienced gestational diabetes are at greater risk of developing type 2 diabetes later.) In fact, gestational diabetes generally stops abruptly when the placenta is delivered.

Does Anything Increase My Risk of Developing Gestational Diabetes?

Any woman can develop gestational diabetes during pregnancy (which is why all women should be screened), but certain factors do increase the risk. These include:

- Obesity
- Family history of diabetes
- Previous pregnancy during which you developed gestational diabetes
- Previously giving birth to a very large infant, a stillborn baby or a child with a birth defect
- Having too much amniotic fluid, a condition called polyhydramnios

When Should I Be Tested for Gestational Diabetes?

In most cases, your obstetrician or nurse midwife will have you undergo a standard screening test for gestational diabetes between the twenty-fourth and twenty-eighth weeks of pregnancy. If you have one or more risk factors, then you may have this test sooner. Also, a routine urine test that shows you have sugar in your urine is another reason to have the screening test earlier.

How Am I Tested for Gestational Diabetes?

There are several types of screening tests, and your health care provider will determine which one is best for you and your medical/family history. Most tests involve drinking a sugary liquid and then having your blood drawn to see how your body—in particular, your pancreas's ability to produce insulin—responds to the sugar load. Depending on the test, you may or may not have to fast ahead of time; also, with some tests, you will have blood drawn just once, but with others, you will have blood drawn several times, at specified intervals. If the results of the first test are abnormal, you may have to be retested. Again, only your health-care provider will know which test, or series of tests, is best for you.

Can Gestational Diabetes Hurt My Baby?

Even though the short answer to this is yes, you should know that gestational diabetes is manageable. Testing for gestational diabetes and, then, if it is present, careful medical and dietary management are key to preventing complications.

You may have heard that women with type 1 diabetes are more likely to have babies with birth defects. Indeed, this is true. However, gestational diabetes is not associated with birth defects. It's easy to understand why. As you have learned, gestational diabetes generally starts toward the end of the second or the beginning of the third trimester, long after baby has finished "sketching in" all of his or her organs and tissues. (After that, baby simply colors in the sketches, or grows in size.)

However, too-high blood sugars in the second and third trimester can cause one big problem: macrosomia, or babies born larger than the healthy average. As you have learned in Chapters One and Two of this book, babies born larger than average are at increased risk for developing certain cancers and also for becoming overweight as they grow into adult life.

Let me explain how higher-than-normal blood sugars can cause baby to grow excessively. When the maternal blood has too much glucose, the pancreas of the fetus senses this. In turn, the fetal pancreas pumps out extra insulin to try to normalize its own blood sugars. Yes, even though the mom has a problem with producing the right amount of or using insulin properly, her baby usually just keeps pumping out the insulin when sugar is present.

Because a baby needs only so much glucose to grow normally, he or she stores the extra as fat. Though the baby needs some fat, he or she doesn't stop storing fat at what might be considered the optimal level. Indeed, the fat pads just keep building up (as they do in anyone who overeats consistently). If gestational diabetes goes untreated, then baby will be born larger than the healthy average, which is called macrosomia (*macro* for "large" and *somia* for "body"). *However, managing blood sugars through careful medical and nutritional therapy can keep baby growing at a healthy rate.*

Gestational diabetes that is not carefully managed and controlled can also cause baby to have blood sugar problems at birth. Remember, if the baby has to cope alone with high blood sugars, he or she will produce larger-than-normal amounts of insulin. At birth, the baby will continue to have a high level of insulin—but he or she no longer has all that extra sugar around. So, the extra insulin acts on all the sugar it can find, sometimes dropping baby's blood sugar at birth. Again, managing your blood sugar levels carefully during pregnancy, if you do develop gestational diabetes, can prevent this complication. Be assured, the blood sugar levels of all babies born to women with gestational diabetes are monitored carefully at birth and for some time after to detect problems—and correct them promptly.

MANAGING GESTATIONAL DIABETES

As I said at the beginning of this chapter, I do not intend for the information in this chapter alone to help you manage gestational diabetes. Indeed, you need the individualized care that only your obstetrician can recommend. You will probably need to see a registered dietitian, who will design your meal plan around your blood sugars and insulin, if you need it. (Not all women with gestational diabetes need insulin.)

Just so you are aware, the facets that may be involved in caring for you and your gestational diabetes include (but are not limited to):

- *Testing your own blood sugars with a home medical device called a blood sugar monitor:* You will be advised what to purchase, how often to test your blood sugars, how to perform the test, and how to respond to certain test results.
- *Following a diet with optimal amounts of carbohydrate and protein and eating on a certain schedule:* Although the menus we have designed in this book may be just fine for you to follow should you develop gestational diabetes, you need to show them to your obstetrician and/or dietitian to determine if they are appropriate for you. They may show you how to adapt our meals, or they may recommend another eating plan. Remember, each woman with gestational diabetes has unique needs.
- *Taking insulin by injection:* Many women with gestational diabetes achieve good blood sugar control by following carefully the diet prescribed for them. In some cases, though, insulin by injection becomes necessary. If this becomes true for you, your health-care providers will help you become familiar with this routine.
- *Having more frequent medical and/or obstetrical checkups:* Your physician may ask you to return more frequently if you develop gestational diabetes. Don't be alarmed. Frequent checkups are in your best interest, as they help detect problems early, before they become significant issues. You may also have serial ultrasound studies, just to make sure the baby is growing at the appropriate rate, and other types of fetal testing just to make sure.

A Final Word

We want the best for you and your baby. Not only do we want you to have a baby who is healthy at birth, but we also want the adult that your baby will become (in the blink of an eye!) to have the lowest possible risk of chronic diseases. By making you aware of gestational diabetes, how to detect it, and the principles of management, we hope all these things will come true.

CHAPTER TEN

Recipes

An Optimal Cooking and Shopping Primer

Preparing the foods that you and baby need throughout your pregnancy—as well as through your life course—requires at least a cursory understanding of healthy cooking and shopping guidelines. Before you delve into the fabulously delicious recipes that Kris developed just for you during your days in waiting, we'd like to walk you through some shopping and cooking basics.

Shopping Basics, Lesson 1

Save precious time in the grocery store and in the kitchen with the following tips:

- Frequent one grocery store, as you'll know where things are, which is a real time saver.
- Most places now offer on-line or catalogue grocery shopping, which is an incredible time saver, and comes with a freshness guarantee. The best part: no schlepping—they deliver to your door.
- Keep a running list posted on the refrigerator door of items used up, including pantry items.
- Design your shopping list according to our menus. Shopping with lists saves time because you don't have to guess about what you should buy, and you'll be less likely to buy foods you shouldn't eat.

- Don't hesitate to buy precut vegetables and bagged salads. Their nutritional quality is still excellent, and they can save you hours of preparation time.
- If the quality of fresh produce in your store is not great, or if you can't shop regularly, feel free to use frozen vegetables and fruits, as their nutritional quality is still very good. They can also be a useful time saver. (Note that frozen foods retain more nutrients than canned foods.)
- Similarly, choose precut stew and stir-fry meat to save time.
- If your cooking time is limited, find the frozen or canned beans in your grocery store and use them instead of cooking from scratch. (We've included a table on legume cooking, in case you are learning to cook your own.)

Shopping Basics, Lesson 2

If you are confused when you step foot into the grocery store, you are not alone. The average grocery store, says the Food Marketing Institute, has over 30,000 items. On top of that, not every grocery store has the same 30,000 items—which means you can encounter thousands more just by shopping in several different stores. That makes finding healthy choices difficult—even intimidating.

As you enter the grocery store, mentally divide it into green-light, yellow-light, and red-light sections:

- Green-light foods represent the healthiest food choices.
- Yellow-light foods are acceptable food choices; they might be higher in total fat or saturated fat, and, in some cases, they're higher in sodium or sugar or lower in fiber. Use these foods with careful planning.
- Red-light foods should be occasional choices, as they are highest in fat or saturated fat compared to products in the green or yellow categories.

Here is additional detail about this configuration:

- Consider the produce section a green-light area. In fact, spend the majority of your grocery store time lingering long over the produce and choosing carefully. The only questionable choices here are coconuts, which are high in saturated fat and should be used sparingly. Fill your cart with enough produce to serve up two vegetables for dinner and for lunch and at least three fruit servings daily. Go for variety by choosing lots of different colors and textures. Orange-red vegetables generally have a different blend of nutrients than that of green leafy types; similarly, berries offer a nutrient mix distinct from that of oranges or pears.

- Regard the dairy section as a yellow-light area, or an area where you need to choose with caution. Opt for lower-fat versions of the dairy foods that offer such great nutrition benefits: low-fat or nonfat yogurt and milk, nonfat cream cheese and sour cream, reduced-fat cheeses (search out those that are 50% fat reduced). Get to know this section well, taking time to read and study labels. Make it a goal to work your way down on fat content of foods found here; for example, if you currently use whole milk, move to 2%, then 1% and eventually to skim milk. Try the same thing with cream cheese and sour creams. Integrating reduced-fat dairy products is a fabulous way to add interesting dimensions and flavors to low-fat, healthy eating. You can also learn to use a mix of dairy foods with reduced fat and fortified soy foods, such as soymilk and soy cheese.

- The meat department is also a yellow-light area. Be aware that processed meats such as sausages and many coldcuts can be very high in fat. Look for skinless poultry and lean red meat trimmed of fat and with little marbling (lines of fat running through the meat).

- You might be surprised to learn that the bakery is a yellow-light area. There's generally a host of delicious, whole-grain foods that are naturally low in fat and high in vitamins and minerals. Go for the nine-grain bagels, whole-wheat bread, rye dinner rolls, and crispbread, for example. But beware the cakes, cookies, and pastries—they are usually a minefield of added sugar and fat.

- Regard packaged and convenience foods as red-light foods. Many are extremely high in sodium and/or fat (especially saturated fat and *trans*-fatty acids.) Although some can be a part of a healthy diet, it is important to read labels very carefully.

Shopping Basics, Lesson 3

Reading and understanding food labels is also an essential part of healthy shopping. We've summarized here two basic tenets that will help you make sense of food labels:

- An item is low in a particular nutrient if it contains 5% or less of the daily value.
- Foods containing 20% or more of the daily value for a nutrient are considered a good source of desirable nutrients (such as fiber) and high in nutrients you need to limit (such as saturated fat).

Cooking Basics

Lesson 1: General Guidelines
Use some of the following cooking suggestions to make gourmet-style food that is still ever so healthy for you and your growing baby:

- Meat, fish, and poultry can be steamed, stir-sizzled (like stir-frying, but use broth instead of oil), roasted, poached, braised, or baked in parchment paper.
- The flavor of dried herbs and nuts is intensified when toasted or roasted. Toss herbs or nuts in a dry nonstick sauté pan over medium heat for 3 to 4 minutes until lightly toasted. (Be careful with pine nuts; they need less than 1 minute to cook.)
- Adding fresh herbs to warmed olive oil adds extra flavor.
- Juices or flavored vinegars mixed with olive oil reduce the amount of fat used in cooking and add a special taste to your dish.
- To cut down on high-calorie ingredients, use no-calorie extracts, such as coconut and rum extracts, in your recipe.
- High-fat ingredients can be substituted with lower-fat alternatives. You can use Canadian bacon or turkey bacon for regular bacon in recipes.
- Cut high-fat, high-calorie ingredients, such as nuts or olives, into smaller pieces. They will spread more evenly throughout the food, allowing you to use less but get the same level of flavor.
- Using the most intense flavor of a food or ingredient, such as extra-virgin olive oil rather than virgin, or kosher or sea salt rather than regular salt, allows you to use less without losing flavor.

- Using an olive oil spray to grease cooking pans allows you to use less than you would use greasing them the traditional way. Similarly, substitute regular oil with olive-oil spray and broth or very small amounts of an intensely flavored oil, such as sesame oil, when stir-frying.
- Nonstick cookware and utensils don't require greasing.
- Make homemade soups and stocks the day before eating so you have time to chill them. Any fat they contain will solidify on top and can easily be removed.
- Reduced-fat and fat-free dairy products can be substituted for regular choices (milk, sour cream, cream cheese, yogurt, cheese). You may need to experiment to determine when you can use each and enjoy it in a dish. For example, you may be very happy with fat-free yogurt and sour cream but prefer low-fat cream cheese.
- Lower-fat and fat-free marinades intensify the flavor of many foods, including tempeh and tofu, fish, meats, and vegetables.
- Consult the Orange Cream Fruit Tart recipe on page 327 to learn how to make and use yogurt cheese from nonfat and reduced-fat yogurts. This makes a great substitute for cream cheese, butter, and sour cream.

Lesson 2: How to Cook Legumes

Although you have the choice of using canned, precooked legumes, cooking your own is even healthier, as well as more economical. This guide below helps you learn how to cook your own, detailing how much water to use for each one cup of legumes, as well as how long to cook and the final yield. Remember, you can cook up large batches of legumes and freeze them in individual portions for later use.

Cooking Legumes

Legume (1 cup)	Water	Cooking Time After Soaking	Yield
Black beans	4 cups	1½ hours	2 cups
Black-eyed peas	3 cups	1 hour	2 cups
Chickpeas (garbanzo beans)	4 cups	3 hours	2 cups
Great Northern beans	3½ cups	2 hours	2 cups
Kidney beans	3 cups	1½ hours	2 cups
Lentils	3 cups	45 minutes	2¼ cups
Navy beans	3 cups	2½ hours	2 cups
Pinto beans	3 cups	2½ hours	2 cups
Soybeans	4 cups	3+ hours	2 cups
Split peas	3 cups	45 minutes	2¼ cups

Lesson 3: How to Cook Whole Grains

Adding more whole grains into your diet may seem difficult, often just because we are a society that has stopped using them. The table below lists the amount of water to add to each 1 cup of uncooked grain; it also indicates cooking time and yield. As with legumes, you can freeze cooked grains for later use.

Cooking Whole Grains

Grain (1 cup)	Amount of Water	Cooking Time	Yield
Amaranth	4 cups	15–20 minutes	2 cups
Barley (whole)	3 cups	1 hour, 15 minutes	3½ cups
Brown rice	2 cups	50–60 minutes	3 cups
Buckwheat	2 cups	15 minutes	2½ cups
Millet	3 cups	45 minutes	3½ cups
Quinoa	2 cups	15 minutes	2½ cups
Wheat			
Bulgur wheat	2 cups	15–20 minutes	2½ cups
Cracked wheat	2 cups	25 minutes	2⅓ cups
Whole-wheat berries	3 cups	2 hours	2⅔ cups
Wild rice	3 cups	1 hour plus	4 cups

About Our Recipes

The scores of delicious recipes Kris Napier has created especially for pregnant (and soon-to-be pregnant) women are listed in this chapter in the following categories: Muffins, Breads, and Breakfast Cereals; Egg Dishes; Soups and Salads; Pasta Dishes; Vegetarian Main Dishes; Sandwiches and Wraps; Beef, Fish, Pork, and Poultry; Vegetables and Side Dishes; and Desserts, Smoothies, Shakes, and Snacks. At the beginning of each section, we've provided a list of all the recipes included in that section so you can see at a glance if the one you are looking for is there. If it's not, just check the Index (page 361) to find out exactly which page it is on.

Now, on to the best part: easy-to-prepare but gourmet-tasting recipes for you and baby!

Enjoy!

Muffins, Breads, and Breakfast Cereals

Apple Oatmeal

Cooking oats with milk makes them fabulously creamy and also more nutritious. Adding the apple, wheat germ, and brown sugar boosts the flavor volume a few notches.

½ cup uncooked oats
1 cup skim milk
1 apple, sliced (with peel)
1 tablespoon wheat germ
1 teaspoon brown sugar

1. In microwave-safe bowl or saucepan, mix oats, skim milk, apple, wheat germ, and brown sugar.
2. Cook according to package directions for the brand of oats you have chosen.

Preparation time: 5 minutes

Cooking time: Variable, depending on what type of oats you use

Nutrition Information per Serving:
365 calories, 17 g protein, 68 g carbohydrates, 9 g fiber,
4 g fat, 10% calories from fat, 0.28 mg vitamin B_6, 50 mcg folic acid,
339 mg calcium, 3 mg iron, 3 mg zinc

Banana Chocolate Chip Muffins

YIELD: 24 MUFFINS

These muffins freeze well for a quick breakfast or snack later, so don't worry about making too many.

½ cup light olive oil
½ cup applesauce
1½ cups sugar
4 egg whites
4 ripe bananas, mashed (about 1¾ cups mashed)
1 kiwi, peeled and mashed
½ cup nonfat plain yogurt
2 cups all-purpose flour
1¾ cups whole-wheat flour
½ cup wheat germ
1 teaspoon baking soda
1 teaspoon baking powder
¼ teaspoon salt
6 ounces minimorsel semisweet chocolate chips
1 cup milled flax seed
Olive oil spray

1. Preheat the oven to 350° Fahrenheit.
2. In a large bowl, cream together olive oil, applesauce, sugar, egg whites, mashed bananas, and mashed kiwi.
3. Add the remaining ingredients, except chocolate chips; mix them well.
4. Blend in the chocolate chips.
5. Coat 24 muffin tins with the olive oil spray. Fill the muffin tins about ⅔ to ¾ full.
6. Bake the muffins for 20 to 30 minutes, or until a knife inserted into a muffin middle comes out clean.

Preparation time: 15 minutes

Cooking time: 20 to 30 minutes

Nutrition Information per Serving (1 muffin):
250 calories, 5 g protein, 41 g carbohydrates, 4 g fiber,
9 g fat, 31% calories from fat, 0.15 mg vitamin B_6, 24 mcg folic acid,
29 mg calcium, 1 mg iron, 0 mg zinc

Cinnamon-Maple Brown Rice and Raisins

YIELD: 2 SERVINGS

Brown rice is a great food that is loaded with nutrition but is too often ignored. Kris's grandma used to make rice and raisins for breakfast with left-over white rice, which she has recreated with the brown, more nutritious version. Kris uses one of her favorite flavoring secrets: cooking rice with tea bags adds flavor without the usual salt. Make up a big batch of the rice to have on hand; you can also freeze it, once cooked, in individual-size servings.

⅔ cup water
⅓ cup uncooked brown rice
2 orange spice tea bags
½ cup reduced-fat, plain, fortified soymilk, or substitute
     skim milk
¼ cup slivered almonds
½ cup raisins
1 teaspoon cinnamon
1 tablespoon real maple syrup

1. Bring the water to a boil. Add the brown rice and tea bags; stir. Reduce the heat to a simmer. Cook the brown rice per package directions until it is cooked. Remove the teabags. The rice can be cooked the night before and refrigerated until morning.
2. Stir in the soymilk, almonds, raisins, cinnamon, and maple syrup; heat the mix through over low heat. Serve.

Preparation time: 5 minutes

Cooking time: Variable, according to brown rice used

Nutrition Information per Serving:

385 calories, 9 g protein, 67 g carbohydrates, 5 g fiber,
11 g fat, 24% calories from fat, 0.27 mg vitamin B_6, 29 mcg folic acid,
133 mg calcium, 2 mg iron, 2 mg zinc

Corny Cornbread

YIELD: 6 SERVINGS (THIS RECIPE DOUBLES WELL)

Everyone will love this healthy version of cornbread!

    Olive oil spray
    ¼ cup nonfat plain yogurt
    ¼ cup light olive oil
    1 egg white
    ½ cup stone-ground yellow cornmeal
    ½ cup flour
    1 ¼ teaspoons baking powder
    2 tablespoons sugar
    ½ cup frozen corn, defrosted
    Optional: 1 or 2 jalapeno peppers, seeded and chopped
       finely

1. Preheat the oven to 400° Fahrenheit. Coat 6 muffin tins with the olive oil spray.
2. In a large bowl, mix the yogurt, olive oil, and egg white with a large spoon. Add the cornmeal, flour, baking powder, and sugar; mix them well with a spoon just until blended. If you are adding jalapeno peppers, stir them in.
3. Stir in the corn.
4. Divide the batter between 6 muffin tins. Bake the muffins on the bottom shelf of the oven 13 to 15 minutes, or until the edges are browned and the muffins are firm to the touch in the middle.

Preparation time: 10 minutes

Cooking time: 15 minutes

Nutrition Information per Serving:
197 calories, 4 g protein, 25 g carbohydrates, 2 g fiber,
9 g fat, 43% calories from fat, 0.08 mg vitamin B_6, 29 mcg folic acid,
16 mg calcium, 1 mg iron, 0 mg zinc

Craisin–Raisin Oatmeal

Yield: 1 Serving

Another tasty version of oh-so-creamy oatmeal.

½ cup uncooked oats
1 cup skim milk
¼ cup dried cranberries (Craisin brand)
2 tablespoons raisins

1. Mix all ingredients in a microwave-safe container or small saucepan.
2. Cook according to the package directions of the brand of oats you are using, stirring once or twice during cooking time.

Preparation time: 5 minutes

Cooking time: Variable, according to the brand of oats you are using

Nutrition Information per Serving:

393 calories, 16 g protein, 77 g carbohydrates, 7 g fiber,
4 g fat, 8% calories from fat, 0.20 mg vitamin B_6, 26 mcg folic acid,
336 mg calcium, 2 mg iron, 2 mg zinc

Cranberry Pumpkin Muffins

YIELD: 2 DOZEN MUFFINS

Pumpkin is such a wonderful food, loaded with copper, zinc, and vitamin A. It also tastes so sweet when blended with just the right ingredients, as this recipe does. Make a batch of muffins and freeze them individually for snacks and later meals. The dried cranberries are a delightful color and taste addition. Kris has made these much lower in fat than the typical muffin by using a mixture of olive oil and applesauce.

Olive oil spray
⅓ cup light olive oil
⅓ cup applesauce
2⅔ cups sugar
8 egg whites
1 can (15-ounce) unsweetened pumpkin, or 15 ounces
    fresh, cooked pumpkin, puréed
⅔ cup nonfat plain yogurt
1 cup wheat germ
2⅓ cups all purpose flour
2 teaspoons baking soda
½ teaspoon baking powder
1 teaspoon ground cinnamon
1 teaspoon ground cloves
1 cup dried cranberries (Craisins)

1. Preheat the oven to 350° Fahrenheit. Spray 24 muffin tins with olive oil spray or line with muffin papers.
2. Combine the olive oil, applesauce, sugar, egg whites, pumpkin, yogurt, and wheat germ in a large bowl; mix everything at medium speed with an electric mixer or beat by hand until all ingredients are well blended.
3. Add the remainder of ingredients, except dried cranberries, and mix just until flour is blended in. Stir in the dried cranberries.
4. Fill muffin tins ⅔ full; bake for 20 to 30 minutes or until a knife inserted into the middle of a muffin comes out clean.

Preparation time: 15 minutes

Cooking time: 20 to 30 minutes

Nutrition Information per Serving (1 muffin):
203 calories, 4 g protein, 40 g carbohydrates, 2 g fiber,
3 g fat, 15% calories from fat, 0.02 mg vitamin B_6, 21 mcg folic acid,
22 mg calcium, 1 mg iron, 0 mg zinc

Herbed Garlic Cheese Bread

YIELD: 2 SERVINGS

Who doesn't love fat-laden garlic cheese bread? Now you can enjoy it more frequently with this recipe that slashes the fat!

> 4 ounces (2 pieces) crusty Italian bread
> 1 tablespoon extra-virgin olive oil
> 1 tablespoon crushed garlic (bought in a jar, or finely
>   chopped fresh garlic)
> 1 teaspoon Italian seasoning
> 1 tablespoon plus 1 teaspoon fat-free parmesan cheese
> ¼ cup 50% reduced fat cheddar cheese

1. Slice bread lengthwise.
2. In a small bowl, mix the olive oil, garlic, Italian seasoning, and parmesan cheese. Spread this mixture evenly over both pieces of bread.
3. Sprinkle cheddar cheese evenly over the top.
4. Place the bread under a broiler until the cheese melts.

Preparation time: 5 minutes

Cooking time: 5 minutes

Nutrition Information per Serving:
265 calories, 11 g protein, 31 g carbohydrates, 2 g fiber,
10 g fat, 35% calories from fat, 0.09 mg vitamin B_6, 56 mcg folic acid,
120 mg calcium, 2 mg iron, 1 mg zinc

Where to Find Fat-Free Parmesan Cheese

Fat-free parmesan cheese is easy to find, although it isn't found in the same place in every grocery store. In some stores, you'll find it in the dairy case, next to the other shaker containers of parmesan. In some stores, it's in the pasta aisle, by the sauce. Don't hesitate to ask for it; it's widely available in several brands.

Karin's Müsli

YIELD: 1 SERVING

This is Karin's breakfast almost every day. Yes, you can eat oats without cooking them. They actually are already partially cooked when you buy them; you just cook them further when you make oatmeal. They're fabulously healthy, especially combined with all these power nuts and dried fruits. If you enjoy this, you can mix up several servings of the dates, walnuts, oats, cinnamon, and raisins and store them in a plastic or glass container in the refrigerator. Then, measure out one portion and add the raspberries and milk.

> 2 dates
> 2 tablespoons walnuts
> ⅓ cup dry rolled oats (uncooked oatmeal)
> ¼ teaspoon cinnamon
> 2 tablespoons raisins
> 1 cup fresh or frozen raspberries
> ½ cup skim milk

1. Chop the dates and walnuts and place them in large cereal bowl.
2. Add dry rolled oats, cinnamon, and raisins; mix everything well.
3. Add the raspberries and skim milk and mix well. Allow the müsli to stand for 5 to 10 minutes before you eat it so that the oats soften.

Preparation time: 5 minutes

Cooking time: none

Nutrition Information per Serving:

411 calories, 14 g protein, 69 g carbohydrates, 14 g fiber,
12 g fat, 24% calories from fat, 0.32 mg vitamin B_6, 60 mcg folic acid,
223 mg calcium, 3 mg iron, 3 mg zinc

Mandarin Breakfast Broil

YIELD: 1 SERVING

Finding interesting breakfast meals can be tough. This is a twist on the old cottage-cheese-and-fruit routine; you're sure to love it.

> ½ cup fat-free extra-calcium cottage cheese
> 1 whole-wheat English muffin
> 1 cup mandarin orange sections, canned in juice, drained
>   and patted dry
> 1 teaspoon brown sugar
> 1 teaspoon cinnamon (or to taste)

1. Open the English muffin and place ¼ cup of cottage cheese on each half.
2. Place half of the mandarin oranges on each half.
3. Sprinkle both halves with brown sugar and cinnamon and broil for 3 to 4 minutes, or just until sugar starts to bubble.

Preparation time: 5 minutes

Cooking time: 5 minutes

Nutrition Information per Serving:
329 calories, 20 g protein, 63 g carbohydrates, 7 g fiber,
2 g fat, 4% calories from fat, 0.22 mg vitamin B_6, 40 mcg folic acid,
474 mg calcium, 3 mg iron, 2 mg zinc

Egg Dishes

Breakfast Strata

YIELD: 4 SERVINGS

This is a breakfast egg dish that's great as leftovers, hot or cold.

8 egg whites
1 cup skim milk
¼ teaspoon salt
3 slices whole-wheat bread, cut into chunks
2 ounces lean Canadian bacon or very lean ham
½ cup chopped red bell peppers
½ cup chopped green bell peppers
½ cup chopped onions
10-ounce package frozen chopped spinach, thawed and
  drained
1 ounce cheddar cheese

1. Beat the egg whites, skim milk, and salt in a small bowl; set aside.
2. In a medium-size casserole dish, toss the bread chunks, Canadian bacon, chopped peppers, chopped onions, and spinach.
3. Pour the milk–egg mixture over the top, then fold in in.
4. Bake the strata for 30 minutes, uncovered, at 350° Fahrenheit.
5. Sprinkle the cheddar cheese over the top. Bake the strata an additional 10 minutes, or until the cheese bubbles.
6. Let the strata stand 15 minutes before cutting it.

Preparation time: 10 minutes

Cooking time: 40 minutes

Nutrition Information per Serving:
196 calories, 19 g protein, 21 g carbohydrates, 5 g fiber,
5 g fat, 22% calories from fat, 0.35 mg vitamin B_6, 114 mcg folic acid,
233 mg calcium, 3 mg iron, 2 mg zinc

Cheesy Mushroom Omelet

YIELD: 1 SERVING

A great omelet!

    Olive oil spray
    2 egg whites
    ½ cup chopped green onion
    ½ cup thinly sliced mushrooms
    Freshly ground black pepper to taste
    2 slices (about 1⅓ ounces) cheddar flavored soy cheese (or
        1⅓ ounces 50% reduced-fat cheddar cheese)

1. Spray a small nonstick pan evenly with olive oil spray; heat it over low heat.
2. Lightly and briefly beat the egg whites, without creating a foam; pour them into the pan.
3. Just when the eggs start to congeal, sprinkle them with the green onions, mushrooms, and black pepper.
4. Cover the omelet with cheese slices.
5. Cover the pan and allow the omelet to cook slowly until the cheese is melted.
6. Slide the omelet out of the pan and fold it over.

Preparation time: 10 minutes

Cooking time: 5 minutes

Nutrition Information per Serving:

141 calories, 17 g protein, 7 g carbohydrates, 2 g fiber,
4 g fat, 29% calories from fat, 0.08 mg vitamin B_6, 44 mcg folic acid,
42 mg calcium, 1 mg iron, 1 mg zinc

Where to Find Soy Cheese

Nearly all grocery stores carry soy cheese now. Taste-test various brands, because some are better than others. Many brands come in several flavors, from mozzarella to cheddar. I find that the types that come individually wrapped are better than those found in a large hunk.

Creamed Eggs

YIELD: 2 SERVINGS

This was Kris's husband's grandmother's favorite egg dish; of course, she used cream and put the egg yolk on the top. Here, Kris has left that off and made this dish incredibly healthy and full of protein. It also goes down well for breakfast, lunch, or dinner when you are not feeling well.

10 egg whites
1 tablespoon light olive oil
1¼ cups skim milk
2 tablespoons all-purpose flour
⅛ teaspoon salt
⅛ teaspoon black pepper
2 teaspoons sugar
2 whole-wheat English muffins

1. Hard-boil the eggs and separate the whites from the yolks. Chop the whites and set them aside.
2. Heat the oil over medium to low heat in a nonstick pan. As the oil heats, mix the milk and flour in a small bowl until the mixture is free of lumps.
3. When the oil has heated, add the flour–milk mixture, stirring it with a wooden spoon or a whisk suitable for a nonstick pan. Stir until the mixture has thickened. Add freshly ground black pepper, sugar, and salt.
4. Remove the mixture from heat and fold in the egg whites. Serve the dish over whole-grain toast or whole-grain English muffin.

Preparation time: 10 minutes

Cooking time: 10 minutes

Nutrition Information per Serving:
365 calories, 29 g protein, 46 g carbohydrates, 5 g fiber,
7 g fat, 18% calories from fat, 0.18 mg vitamin B$_6$, 52 mcg folic acid,
375 mg calcium, 2 mg iron, 2 mg zinc

Egg–Cheese Breakfast Stack

Yield: 1 Serving

This protein-loaded breakfast is a great way to get your energy level up. It also tastes fabulous!

> 2 eggs
> 1 whole-wheat English muffin
> 2 ounces low-fat cheese
> 1 teaspoon margarine

1. Poach the eggs.
2. Toast the English muffin and spread each half with margarine.
3. Place 1 slice of cheese and then the poached egg on each half of the hot muffin.

Preparation time: 10 minutes

Cooking time: 5 minutes

Nutrition Information per Serving:

418 calories, 33 g protein, 30 g carbohydrates, 4 g fiber,

19 g fat, 41% calories from fat, 0.27 mg vitamin B_6, 68 mcg folic acid,

612 mg calcium, 3 mg iron, 4 mg zinc

Ham and Mushroom Quiche

YIELD: 4 SERVINGS

Although this makes an easy dinner, the leftovers also make a great breakfast, hot or cold.

> 1 cup egg substitute (or 8 egg whites)
> 1 cup skim milk
> ¼ teaspoon salt
> ¼ teaspoon black pepper
> 9-inch ready-made pie crust
> 6 ounces lean ham
> ¼ pound mushrooms, sliced
> 3 ounces low-fat Swiss cheese

1. Preheat the oven to 375° Fahrenheit.
2. Mix the egg substitute, skim milk, salt, and pepper in small mixing bowl; set the mixture aside.
3. Place the ham, mushrooms, and cheese in the unbaked pie crust.
4. Pour the egg–milk mixture over the top.
5. Bake the quiche at 375° Fahrenheit for 30 to 40 minutes, or until its center doesn't jiggle.

Preparation time: 10 minutes

Cooking time: 30 to 40 minutes

Nutrition Information per Serving:
329 calories, 24 g protein, 23 g carbohydrates, 1 g fiber,
15 g fat, 42% calories from fat, 0.10 mg vitamin B_6, 23 mcg folic acid,
321 mg calcium, 2 mg iron, 2 mg zinc

Individual Pumpkin Pie Custards

YIELD: 8 SERVINGS

This recipe eliminates the crust, which is by nature high in fat. You'll enjoy this healthier version and never miss the crust—I promise! Pumpkin pie custards make a great high-protein snack and an interesting breakfast food.

> 15-ounce can pumpkin (or 15 ounces fresh, cooked
>   pumpkin, puréed)
> ¾ cup granulated sugar
> 1 teaspoon ground cinnamon
> ½ teaspoon ground ginger
> ¼ teaspoon ground cloves
> ½ cup liquid egg substitute
> 12 ounces low-fat, plain, fortified soymilk (or 12 ounces
>   evaporated skim milk)
> Olive oil spray
> *Optional:* 1 cup low-fat frozen whipped topping (can
>   substitute vanilla low-fat yogurt)

1. Preheat the oven to 350° Fahrenheit.
2. Combine all the ingredients in large mixing bowl. Stir them with a spoon or whisk until well combined.
3. Spray 8 small custard cups with the olive oil spray. Divide the mixture evenly between cups.
4. Bake the custards for about 20 minutes, or until a knife inserted into the middle of one custard comes out clean.
5. Serve slightly warm with 2 tablespoons whipped topping on each serving.

Preparation time: 10 minutes

Cooking time: 20 minutes

Nutrition Information per Serving:
148 calories, 4 g protein, 28 g carbohydrates, 2 g fiber,
2 g fat, 14% calories from fat, 0.03 mg vitamin B_6, 16 mcg folic acid,
62 mg calcium, 1 mg iron, 0 mg zinc

Western Omelet

YIELD: 1 SERVING

A variety of veggies in this tasty omelet help to sneak in more of the nutrients you and your baby crave!

Olive oil spray
3 egg whites (or ¾ cup liquid egg substitute)
⅛ teaspoon salt
½ cup chopped mushrooms
½ cup chopped tomatoes
¼ cup chopped green onions

1. Spray a small nonstick pan with the olive oil spray and heat it over medium heat.
2. Beat the egg whites slightly, add the salt, and pour the whites into the pan.
3. Just as the eggs start to congeal (they will start to turn white), add the vegetables.
4. Cover the pan, turn down the heat to low, and cook the omelet 5 to 7 minutes, or until the egg white is totally cooked.
5. Slide the omelet out of the pan and fold it.

Preparation time: 5 minutes

Cooking time: 10 minutes

Nutrition Information per Serving:
84 calories, 12 g protein, 8 g carbohydrates, 2 g fiber,
0 g fat, 4% calories from fat, 0.10 mg vitamin B_6, 22 mcg folic acid,
11 mg calcium, 1 mg iron, 1 mg zinc

Soups and Salads

SOUPS

SALADS

Cream of Broccoli Soup

Yield: 4 Servings

This gentle-on-the-stomach, yet flavorful soup is a powerhouse of vitamins and minerals. Be sure to see page 92 about different types of bouillon and why using different versions is important to your health.

8 cups cut-up broccoli (about 2 large heads with stems) or
    8 cups frozen broccoli pieces
1 cup water
1 tablespoon prepared yellow mustard
1 tablespoon chicken bouillon granules
1 tablespoon very low sodium chicken bouillon granules
1 tablespoon extra-virgin olive oil
3 cloves garlic (chopped)
2 cups chopped Vidalia onion
Freshly ground black pepper as desired (about ¼ teaspoon)
2 cups skim milk
8 ounces fat-free cream cheese
3 tablespoons flour
2 ounces grated sharp cheddar cheese

1. Combine the broccoli, water, mustard, and bouillon in a large heavy pot; cover it and bring the mixture to a boil. Reduce heat and simmer the soup until the broccoli is fork tender but still brilliant green.
2. Meanwhile, heat the olive oil, garlic, onion, and black pepper over low heat in a large skillet, sautéeing for 5 minutes.
3. In 2 or 3 batches, process cooked onion and garlic, cooked broccoli with cooking liquid, milk, cream cheese, flour, and cheddar cheese in a food processor or blender. Return the soup to the pot and reheat over medium-low heat, stirring until it is hot and thick.

Preparation time: 15 minutes

Cooking time: 15 minutes

Nutrition Information per Serving:
264 calories, 21 g protein, 25 g carbohydrates, 4 g fiber,
10 g fat, 33% calories from fat, 0.35 mg vitamin B_6, 140 mcg folic acid,
434 mg calcium, 2 mg iron, 2 mg zinc

Taste of Summer Vegetable Lentil Soup

YIELD: 5 SERVINGS

Try this light and refreshing lentil soup recipe—the tastes of lemon and basil, together with lots of summer vegetables, will remind you of summer all year long. This is a great way to include folic acid-rich lentils in your diet, even through the warm weather.

2 tablespoons light olive oil
1 cup chopped onion (about 2 small onions)
2 cloves garlic, chopped
28-ounce can crushed tomatoes
1 cup uncooked lentils
¼ cup uncooked black beans
2 teaspoons vegetable bouillon granules (or 2 cubes)
3 cups water
½ teaspoon chili powder
½ teaspoon ground cumin
¼ teaspoon ground black pepper
¼ cup plus 2 tablespoons chopped fresh basil, divided
¼ cup plus 2 tablespoons lemon juice, divided
1 pound baby spinach leaves
½ pound yellow zucchini, sliced
1 green pepper, chopped
1 red pepper, chopped

Garnish:
2 medium tomatoes, chopped
5 tablespoons fat-free sour cream

1. Heat the olive oil in a large soup kettle, with the onions and garlic, over low heat.
2. Sauté 5 minutes, or until the onions are transparent.
3. Add the crushed tomatoes, lentils, black beans, bouillon, water, chili powder, cumin, pepper, 2 tablespoons basil, and 2 tablespoons lemon juice. Simmer the soup, uncovered, for 40 minutes.

(continued)

4. Add the remaining basil and lemon juice, spinach, zucchini, and green pepper; simmer the soup 20 minutes. Serve it garnished with chopped tomatoes and sour cream if desired.

Preparation time: 15 minutes

Cooking time: 60 minutes

Nutrition Information per Serving:

330 calories, 20 g protein, 53 g carbohydrates, 21 g fiber,
7 g fat, 17% calories from fat, 0.80 mg vitamin B_6, 350 mcg folic acid,
167 mg calcium, 8 mg iron, 3 mg zinc

Vegetarian Chili

YIELD: 6 SERVINGS

I hope you try the textured vegetable protein (TVP) in this recipe, as it is a good source of copper, iron, and zinc, and other nutrients you need. See the note on page 244 about how to find it. It cooks up like hamburger and picks up the flavor of everything you have cooked it with. Kris's family still thinks it is hamburger! The leftovers freeze well for quick meals later.

2 tablespoons extra-virgin olive oil
4 cloves garlic, minced
2 onions, chopped (about 2 cups)
¾ cup textured vegetable protein (TVP, a soy protein
    available in health-food stores)
4 stalks celery, chopped (about 2 cups)
2 16-ounce cans dark red kidney beans
28-ounce can crushed tomatoes
14.5-ounce can diced tomatoes
2 teaspoons sugar
1 teaspoon dried sweet basil
1 teaspoon dried oregano
1 tablespoon chili powder
1 teaspoon salt
1 tablespoon garlic powder
¼ teaspoon ground black pepper
1 green bell pepper, chopped
1 red bell pepper, chopped
1 yellow bell pepper, chopped
1 orange bell pepper, chopped

1. Add the olive oil to a heavy soup kettle, and heat it over low heat; add the garlic, onions, and TVP and sauté them 5 to 7 minutes, without burning them.
2. Add the remainder of ingredients, except the bell peppers. Reduce heat and simmer the mixture, covered, for 45 minutes, allowing flavors to reach their peak.

(*continued*)

3. Stir in the chopped peppers. Turn off the heat and allow the chili to sit for 10 minutes, until its heat softens the peppers slightly but still leaves them crunchy.

Preparation time: 15 minutes

Cooking time: 60 minutes

Nutrition Information per Serving:
313 calories, 18 g protein, 52 g carbohydrates, 18 g fiber,
6 g fat, 16% calories from fat, 0.61 mg vitamin B_6, 168 mcg folic acid,
166 mg calcium, 6 mg iron, 2 mg zinc

About Textured Vegetable Protein

Textured vegetable protein (TVP) is a soy protein available in health-food stores or the frozen-foods section of your grocery store. It may be called "veggie crumbles" or something similar when frozen. If you can't find TVP, substitute ½ pound ground turkey or sirloin; brown first and pat out extra oil with paper towels.

Arugula with Basil–Balsamic Dressing

YIELD: 2 SERVINGS

Kris loves to use arugula whenever possible because it is one of the few vegetable sources of omega-3 fatty acids, those oh-so-healthy fats that are usually found in fish. It has an exciting peppery flavor I think you'll love. She's also used flaxseed in this recipe, which blends extremely well with the flavors of basil and balsamic vinegar and also adds omega-3 fatty acids. At a leading spa, she demonstrated how to make this salad, and her students asked if they could lick their plates!

3 cloves garlic, minced

8 large fresh basil leaves, chopped

⅓ cup balsamic vinegar

1 tablespoon sugar

½ teaspoon extra-virgin olive oil

Freshly ground black pepper

2 medium tomatoes, thinly sliced

¼ Vidalia onion (or any other sweet variety), thinly sliced
    and separated into rings (omit these if they bother your
    stomach)

4 cups arugula, washed and patted dry

2 tablespoons milled flaxseed

2 cups cooked black beans (see cooking instructions—
    "Cooking Legumes"—on page 218, or use canned beans
    if you're short of time)

1. In a shallow glass container, mix the garlic, basil, vinegar, sugar, oil, and ground pepper.
2. Add the tomatoes and onion to the vinegar mixture.
3. Marinate the mixture at room temperature for 3 hours or overnight in the refrigerator.
4. Divide the arugula between two plates; top each pile with half the dressing mixture.

(continued)

5. Sprinkle 1 tablespoon of the flaxseed and 1 cup of the black beans on each serving.

Preparation time: 10 minutes

Marinade Time: 3 hours

Nutrition Information per Serving:
358 calories, 18 g protein, 62 g carbohydrates, 18 g fiber,
6 g fat, 15% calories from fat, 0.20 mg vitamin B_6, 61 mcg folic acid,
171 mg calcium, 7 mg iron, 0 mg zinc

Flaxseed: Why It's Healthy and Where to Get It

Flaxseed is one of the best kept health secrets: full of minerals, omega-3 fatty acids, and fiber, as well as phytochemicals that help prevent cancer and heart disease. Many stores now carry it, but you may have to look in a health-food store. You can buy it whole or milled (ground). If you buy the whole-seed version, just grind it in a coffee grinder. The body cannot break down the whole flax seed, so it just passes through the body unabsorbed. Store flaxseed in the refrigerator in a tightly sealed container.

About Black Beans

You can purchase black beans already cooked in a can, which makes this dish (and other salads) very easy. If you use the canned version, just drain and rinse to get some of the salt off. If you'd like to cook your own, refer to "Cooking Legumes" on page 218 for how to do so. Note that you can cook large batches of beans and then freeze them in individual-size portions for later. They can be stored in the refrigerator for up to 3 days.

Celery and Apple Salad

YIELD: 2 SERVINGS

One of my favorite carry-to-work salads, this slightly sweet salad satisfies a sweet tooth—as well as the nutrition needs of both a mom and her baby. The paprika adds color and just a gentle little zip.

> 2 tablespoons low-fat vanilla yogurt
> 1 tablespoon honey
> 1 tablespoon lemon juice
> ⅛ teaspoon salt
> ¼ teaspoon paprika
> 1 Granny Smith apple
> 2 stalks celery, with leaves, cleaned and chopped
> 2 tablespoons dried cranberries
> 10 dried apricot halves, chopped
> 2 cups arugula, cleaned and chopped

1. In a small mixing bowl, whisk together the yogurt, honey, lemon juice, salt, and paprika.
2. Wash and core the apple (leave the peel on), then cut it into bite-size pieces.
3. Toss the apple with the sauce, which keeps it from browning and also distributes the flavor nicely.
4. Fold in the chopped celery, cranberries, and chopped apricots.
5. Place half of the salad on 1 cup of arugula leaves. If you are carrying this to work, place the cleaned, dry arugula leaves in a plastic bag and add them only when it's time to eat.

Preparation time: 10 minutes

Cooking time: none

Nutrition Information per Serving:
216 calories, 3 g protein, 55 g carbohydrates, 5 g fiber,
1 g fat, 3% calories from fat, 0.15 mg vitamin B_6, 36 mcg folic acid,
98 mg calcium, 2 mg iron, 1 mg zinc

Cucumber Salad

YIELD: 2 SERVINGS

This stores well in the refrigerator, so feel free to double or triple this recipe.

1 English cucumber, sliced thinly with peel (about 3 cups)
½ cup plain low-fat yogurt
16 fresh mint leaves, chopped (about 2 tablespoons), or 1
 teaspoon dried mint leaves
⅛ teaspoon salt
1 tablespoon rice wine vinegar
2 teaspoons honey

1. Place the mint leaves in a small mixing bowl; whisk in the yogurt, salt, rice wine vinegar, and honey.
2. Fold the cucumbers into the sauce.

Preparation time: 5 minutes.

Cooking time: none

Nutrition Information per Serving:
94 calories, 4 g protein, 18 g carbohydrates, 1 gram fiber,
1 gram fat, 11% calories from fat, 0.1 mg vitamin B$_6$, 27 mcg folic acid,
137 mg calcium, 1 mg iron, 1 mg zinc

Cheddar Cheese–Brazil Nut Salad

YIELD: 2 SERVINGS

This is one of the most interesting salads Kris has ever invented. She wanted to put these ingredients together for the nutrients they provide, and then she figured out a way to make them taste good—so good you'll want to make it every day. The sharp cheddar cheese is high in flavor but also in fat, which is why it's combined with fat-free cottage cheese. Brazil nuts are a great source of selenium and zinc, often difficult-to-get nutrients. Enjoy!

> 1 tablespoon balsamic vinegar
> 1 tablespoon extra-virgin olive oil
> 1 tablespoon Dijon mustard
> 1 teaspoon honey
> Provençal Herbs, as desired (see recipe page 91)
> 4 cups chopped or torn romaine lettuce
> 1 red bell pepper, chopped
> 1 yellow bell pepper, chopped
> ½ cup fat-free extra-calcium cottage cheese
> 2 ounces (½ cup) sharp cheddar cheese
> 8 large Brazil nuts, sliced or chopped
> ¼ cup fat-free croutons (purchased, or you can make your
>   own; see next page)

1. In a small bowl or cup, blend the vinegar, olive oil, mustard, and honey; add herbs if desired; set the mixture aside.
2. Place the lettuce and chopped bell peppers in a salad bowl; mix.
3. Add the cottage cheese and cheddar cheese to the salad bowl; sprinkle the salad with the chopped Brazil nuts and croutons.
4. Drizzle the salad with dressing and toss it.

Preparation time: 10 minutes

Cooking time: none

Nutrition Information per Serving:

433 calories, 20 g protein, 27 g carbohydrates, 5 g fiber,
29 g fat, 58% calories from fat, 0.37 mg vitamin B_6, 186 mcg folic acid,
304 mg calcium, 3 mg iron, 2 mg zinc

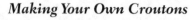

Making Your Own Croutons

Salad croutons add a wonderful crunch that satisfies everyone. Purchased croutons, as well as those in most restaurants, are often loaded with fat. Here's a very healthy alternative:

1. Purchase or make a 12-grain or other whole-grain bread that is not sliced.
2. Slice into 1-inch-thick slices, then cube the slices. (You can cube four or five slices at once to save time).
3. Sprinkle the cubes with garlic powder or other herbs or spices of your choosing (use fresh or dried).
4. Spray a 9" x 13" cookie sheet with olive-oil spray. Place the bread cubes on the cookie sheet and spread them out.
5. Place the cookie sheet in a cold oven and then turn the oven to 450° Fahrenheit. Bake the croutons for approximately 15 minutes, or until they are crisp and slightly browned. Turn them over once or twice during cooking.
6. Allow the croutons to cool and then place them in an airtight container and store them in the refrigerator. You can turn a whole loaf of whole-grain bread into croutons and store them for later use.

Lentil Salad

YIELD: 1 SERVING

An exceptionally easy, high-protein, high-nutrient salad that is a meal in itself.

>   1 cup fresh spinach, chopped
>   1 cup romaine lettuce, chopped
>   1 tomato, chopped
>   1 cup cooked lentils (see "Lesson 2: How to Cook
>   Legumes" about canned beans, on page 218; use canned
>   or make your own)
>   1 tablespoon extra-virgin olive oil
>   1 tablespoon balsamic vinegar

1. In an individual salad bowl, mix together the chopped spinach and romaine lettuce.
2. Top the greens with the chopped tomato, cooked lentils, olive oil, and balsamic vinegar. Add freshly ground black pepper or other favorite herbs if you desire.
3. Toss the salad before serving it.

Preparation time: 5 minutes

Cooking time: none

Nutrition Information per Serving:

410 calories, 21 g protein, 51 g carbohydrates, 19 g fiber,
15 g fat, 33% calories from fat, 0.54 mg vitamin B_6, 511 mcg folic acid,
96 mg calcium, 9 mg iron, 3 mg zinc

Minted Strawberry Salad

YIELD: 1 SERVING

This salad is full of foods that are loaded with essential nutrients for pregnant women and their babies, including copper, folic acid, protein, vitamin C. The flavors blend together beautifully to create a fabulous, gentle melody.

1 cup baby spinach
½ cup chopped tomato
½ cup baby corn
¼ avocado, thinly sliced
1 orange, peeled and separated (peel segments if desired)
½ cup cooked black beans (or canned black beans, rinsed;
    see "Lesson 2: How to Cook Legumes," page 218)
8 large strawberries, sliced

Dressing:
1 tablespoon olive oil
5 strawberries, mashed
16 fresh mint leaves, chopped (about 2 tablespoons), or
    1 teaspoon dried mint leaves

1. Place the spinach on a plate. Top it with the tomatoes and baby corn.
2. Arrange the avocado slices and orange pieces in a circular pattern.
3. Sprinkle the salad with black beans.
4. Top it with the sliced strawberries.
5. Mash the strawberries in a small bowl. Stir in the olive oil and mint. Drizzle the dressing over the salad.

Preparation time: 15 minutes

Cooking time: none

Nutrition Information per Serving:
473 calories, 14 g protein, 66 g carbohydrates, 21 g fiber,
24 g fat, 40% calories from fat, 0.49 mg vitamin B_6, 185 mcg folic acid,
167 mg calcium, 6 mg iron, 1 mg zinc

Nutty Black Bean Salad

YIELD: 1 SERVING

Soy nuts add a great crunch to this healthy salad.

1 cup cooked black beans (see "Cooking Legumes," page 218,
   for how to cook, or buy canned black beans and rinse)
½ cup artichoke hearts, canned in water, chopped
1 carrot, shredded (or 1 cup carrot matchsticks)
2 tablespoons favorite low-fat salad dressing
1 cup chopped spinach
¼ cup soy nuts

1. Combine the black beans, artichoke hearts, and carrots in a small bowl. Add the salad dressing and mix well.
2. Place the mixture on top of the spinach and garnish the salad with soy nuts.

Preparation time: 5 minutes

Cooking time: none

Nutrition Information per Serving:
420 calories, 26 g protein, 66 g carbohydrates, 24 g fiber,
9 g fat, 19% calories from fat, 0.36 mg vitamin B_6, 211 mcg folic acid,
224 mg calcium, 10 mg iron, 2 mg zinc

Nutty Kiwi Salad

Yield: 4 Servings

Kris keeps this in the refrigerator for those times when she needs a complete meal in a hurry or a healthy power snack.

> 6 kiwis, washed and sliced, and each slice quartered
> 1 cup roasted soy nuts (see the information about soy nuts on page 82; you can substitute ½ cup almonds or walnuts)
> 1 cup low-fat lemon yogurt

1. Mix all ingredients.
2. Serve.

Preparation time: 5 minutes

Cooking time: none

Nutrition Information per Serving:
217 calories, 12 g protein, 32 g carbohydrates, 5 g fiber,
6 g fat, 24% calories from fat, 0.16 mg vitamin B_6, 66 mcg folic acid,
163 mg calcium, 1 mg iron, 1 mg zinc

Orange–Spinach Salad

YIELD: 2 SERVINGS

A powerhouse of folic acid, copper, and zinc—and the most fabulous flavor.

1 pound baby spinach leaves
2-ounce can mandarin oranges (packed in juice or light
    syrup), drained, chopped
¼ cup chopped walnuts

Dressing:
4 tablespoons orange juice
1 tablespoon extra-virgin olive oil
½ teaspoon salt
Pepper to taste

1. Wash and dry the spinach, then split it between 2 plates.
2. Top each plateful with half of the mandarin oranges, then sprinkle
   each with 2 tablespoons of walnuts.
3. In a small bowl, whisk together the orange juice, olive oil, salt, and
   pepper.
4. Pour half of the dressing over each salad.

Preparation time: 10 minutes

Cooking time: none

Nutrition Information per Serving:
236 calories, 9 g protein, 17 g carbohydrates, 8 g fiber,
17 g fat, 60% calories from fat, 0.56 mg vitamin B_6, 465 mcg folic acid,
247 mg calcium, 7 mg iron, 2 mg zinc

Poppyseed Salmon Salad

YIELD: 2 SERVINGS

Ever tried bok choy ? It's a delicious Chinese vegetable that is now available in most supermarkets. It combines fabulous flavor and power-packed nutrients with a minimum of calories.

> 1 tomato, chopped
> ¼ cup fat-free poppyseed dressing
> 2 cups canned pink salmon (with bones, but skin removed)
> 1 cup bok choy
> 4 cups spinach

1. In a small bowl, toss the chopped tomato with the poppyseed dressing.
2. Add the salmon and toss.
3. In another small bowl, toss the two greens together.
4. Top them with the salad mixture and serve.

Preparation time: 10 minutes

Cooking time: none

Nutrition Information per Serving:

281 calories, 34 g protein, 14 g carbohydrates, 2 g fiber,
10 g fat, 32% calories from fat, 0.79 mg vitamin B_6, 273 mcg folic acid,
470 mg calcium, 5 mg iron, 2 mg zinc

Quinoa Roasted Red Pepper Salad

YIELD: 2 SERVINGS

Quinoa is a wonderful grain that is underused, just because it seems like such a mystery. You can now find it in most grocery stores, in the grain section, or sometimes in the vegetable aisle, and you can always find it in the health-food store. It is loaded with protein and many minerals that are often hard to find. Besides that, it is so very tasty.

> 1 tablespoon extra-virgin olive oil
> ¼ teaspoon salt
> Freshly ground black pepper to taste
> 1 cup cooked quinoa
> 1 cup French haricot green beans, steamed (or 1 cup
>   frozen green beans, thawed)
> ½ cup frozen corn, thawed
> ½ of 7.25-ounce jar roasted red peppers (not in oil),
>   drained and chopped
> 2 cups chopped romaine lettuce
> 2 cups chopped arugula

1. In a small bowl, blend the olive oil, salt, and pepper. Add the cooked quinoa and toss it.
2. Add the green beans, corn, and chopped red peppers; toss the salad.
3. Place the salad over the chopped greens.

Preparation time: 10 minutes

Cooking time: none

Nutrition Information per Serving:

461 calories, 15 g protein, 76 g carbohydrates, 10 g fiber,
13 g fat, 24% calories from fat, 0.32 mg vitamin B_6, 155 mcg folic acid,
141 mg calcium, 10 mg iron, 4 mg zinc

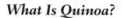

What Is Quinoa?

Pronounced KEEN-wah, quinoa is actually a dried seed from the goosefoot plant, and it's especially high in protein. That's how this salad becomes a meal in itself without beans, fish, or meat. Quinoa is also very high in soluble fiber and in phytochemicals that protect us from disease. Most grocery stores carry it now, or you can buy it in a health-food store. When you cook it, use 2 parts water to 1 part quinoa and simmer it approximately 15 to 20 minutes. You can cook a large batch and freeze it in plastic storage bags in the freezer.

Green Beans . . . and Different Green Beans

Have you ever seen those skinny little green beans in the produce section? Try them. They're haricot beans, a very tender version of regular green beans, and they add immense interest to a salad just because of their slender shape. If you don't want to bother taking the ends off beans (of any sort), then buy any frozen type, thaw and drain it, and use it in **Quinoa Roasted Red Pepper Salad.**

Rainbow Meal Salad

YIELD: 2 SERVINGS

Here's a salad for which Kris has developed two versions. The protein in this one is a very different, sweet version of soy, the green soybean, also called mukimi edamame, or just edamame. Green soybeans are very easy to find, available in most grocery stores in the frozen-foods section (where the other vegetables are). Frozen green soybeans generally come already cooked, and you just have to place them in boiling water for 5 to 6 minutes to heat them. Once cooked, they store well in the freezer. You'll find that their taste is completely different from that of tofu or tempeh.

> 2 teaspoons extra-virgin olive oil
> 4 teaspoons orange juice
> Freshly ground black pepper or fresh herbs of your choice
> 2 cups cooked green soybeans, cooled
> 12 olives, chopped (Kalamata olives are best)
> 1 cup sliced mushrooms
> ½ red pepper, chopped
> ½ yellow pepper, chopped
> 1 cup grated carrots (or carrot matchsticks available in a
>   bag in the produce section)
> 1 cup mesclun greens
> 2 cups chopped spinach
> 2 kiwis, peeled and sliced, then quartered

1. In a large salad bowl, mix the olive oil and orange juice; add the freshly ground black pepper or fresh or dried herbs of your choice (see Karin's favorite herb blend, Provençal Herbs, page 91).
2. Stir in the cooled, cooked green soybeans, chopped olives, and sliced mushrooms. Toss the ingredients to distribute the sauce and herbs well.

(continued)

3. Fold in the chopped peppers and carrots.
4. Place the mixture on a bed of mesclun greens and spinach; garnish with the kiwis.

Preparation time: 15 minutes.

Cooking time: none

Nutrition Information per Serving:
437 calories, 26 g protein, 47 g carbohydrates, 15 g fiber,
20 g fat, 38% calories from fat, 0.51 mg vitamin B_6, 324 mcg folic acid,
359 mg calcium, 8 mg iron, 2 mg zinc

Rainbow Side Salad

YIELD: 2 SERVINGS

Here's the side version of a most eye-appealing and interesting, nutritious salad.

> 2 teaspoons extra virgin olive oil
> 4 teaspoons orange juice
> Freshly ground black pepper or fresh herbs of your choice
> 12 olives, chopped (Kalamata olives are best)
> 1 cup sliced mushrooms
> ½ red pepper, chopped
> ½ yellow pepper, chopped
> 1 cup grated carrots (or carrot matchsticks available in a
>   bag in the produce section)
> 1 cup mesclun greens
> 2 cups chopped spinach
> 2 kiwis, peeled, sliced, and then quartered

1. In a large salad bowl, mix the olive oil and orange juice; add the freshly ground black pepper or fresh or dried herbs of your choice (see Karin's favorite herb blend, Provençal Herbs, page 91).
2. Stir in the chopped olives and sliced mushrooms. Toss the mixture to distribute the sauce and herbs well.
3. Fold in the chopped peppers and carrots.
4. Place the mixture on a bed of mesclun greens and spinach; garnish the salad with kiwis.

Preparation time: 20 minutes

Cooking time: none

Nutrition Information per Serving:
183 calories, 4 g protein, 27 g carbohydrates, 7 g fiber,
8 g fat, 38% calories from fat, 0.40 mg vitamin B_6, 124 mcg folic acid,
98 mg calcium, 3 mg iron, 0.83 mg zinc

Raspberry Asparagus Quinoa Salad

YIELD: 2 SERVINGS

Here's another great way to get some delicious, nutritious quinoa into your diet. This recipe uses one of my favorite tricks, cooking grains with a tea bag instead of salt. The flavor advantage is tremendous! For more information on quinoa, see "What Is Quinoa?" on page 258.

    1 cup water
    1 raspberry tea bag
    ½ teaspoon extra-virgin olive oil
    ½ cup uncooked quinoa
    ½ pound asparagus, with tough ends snapped off
    2 tablespoons raspberry vinegar (or raspberry red wine
       vinegar)
    1 teaspoon extra-virgin olive oil
    2 teaspoons orange marmalade (with rind)
    ⅛ teaspoon salt
    ½ cup chopped red onion
    7.5-ounce can mandarin oranges, packed in juice, drained
       well and patted dry
    4 cups baby spinach
    ¼ cup dried cranberries (Craisins) or ½ cup fresh or frozen
       raspberries
    ½ cup roasted soy nuts or ¼ cup chopped macadamia nuts

1. In a pot, bring the water to a boil with the raspberry tea bag and ½ teaspoon extra-virgin olive oil. Add the quinoa; stir well, cover the pot and reduce the heat to a simmer. Simmer the quinoa mixture 15 minutes.
2. Meanwhile, steam the whole asparagus until it is crisp yet tender. After steaming, rinse the asparagus immediately in icy cold water to stop the cooking and to retain its vivid green color. Slice the asparagus on the diagonal, reserving the tips, and set it aside.
3. Mix together the raspberry vinegar, 1 teaspoon extra-virgin olive oil, orange marmalade, and salt; set the mixture aside.
4. After the quinoa has simmered 15 minutes and soaked up all the liquid, remove the tea bag. Toss the quinoa with the raspberry

vinegar. Fold in the chopped red onion and sliced asparagus, except for the reserved tips. Chill this mixture at least 1 hour in shallow container.

5. After the quinoa has chilled, divide the spinach between 2 plates, and top each with half the quinoa mixture. Garnish with asparagus tips, mandarin oranges, dried cranberries, and roasted soy nuts.

Preparation time: 20 minutes
(including simmering while you are
preparing other ingredients)

Cooling time: 1 hour

Nutrition Information per Serving:
463 calories, 20 g protein, 77 g carbohydrates, 10 g fiber,
12 g fat, 21% calories from fat, 0.63 mg vitamin B_6, 322 mcg folic acid,
155 mg calcium, 7 mg iron, 3 mg zinc

Ready-to-go Fruit Salad

YIELD: 4 SERVINGS

It's great to have fruit all cut up in the refrigerator, especially a combination that supplies many important nutrients. You can keep this about 3 to 4 days in the fridge and enjoy it frequently.

1 kiwi, sliced
1 banana, sliced
1 cup sliced fresh strawberries
1 apple, sliced
2 cups grapes
¼ cup calcium-fortified orange juice
2 tablespoons fresh lemon juice
1 tablespoon sugar

1. Mix the orange juice, lemon juice, and sugar in a small bowl.
2. Toss the mixture with the fruit.

Preparation time: 10 minutes

Cooking time: none

Nutrition Information per Serving:
150 calories, 1 g protein, 38 g carbohydrates, 4 g fiber,
1 g fat, 5% calories from fat, 0.32 mg vitamin B_6, 23 mcg folic acid,
43 mg calcium, 1 mg iron, 0 mg zinc

Rice and Asparagus Salad

YIELD: 1 SERVING

This fun, high-flavor recipe makes a great take-to-work lunch. Remember, you can cook up a big batch of brown rice and store it in the freezer in individual-size portions for when you need it—like to make this dish.

1 cup grated carrots (or carrot matchsticks)
2 tablespoons hulled, roasted sunflower seeds
1 cup long-grain brown rice, cooked
10 asparagus spears, steamed

Dressing:
2 teaspoons lemon juice
2 teaspoons olive oil
1 teaspoon honey

Preparation time: 10 minutes (once rice is cooked)

Cooking time: varies according to directions on rice package

Nutrition Information per Serving:

496 calories, 13 g protein, 73 g carbohydrates, 11 g fiber,
19 g fat, 34% calories from fat, 0.76 mg vitamin B_6, 282 mcg folic acid,
92 mg calcium, 3 mg iron, 3 mg zinc

Rotini Chicken Salad with Peanut Sauce

YIELD: 1 SERVING

A wonderfully interesting pasta salad that meets so many of your nutritional needs. And it tastes better the longer it sits! Store it in the refrigerator for up to 3 days.

1½ tablespoons smooth peanut butter
1½ tablespoons light soy sauce
1 tablespoon sugar
¼ cup chopped fresh cilantro
½ grated large carrot
¼ cup chopped green onions
¾ cup rotini pasta, cooked
3-ounce skinless, boneless chicken breast, cooked, cooled,
  and cubed
1 cup chopped romaine lettuce

1. In a small bowl, mix the peanut butter, soy sauce, sugar, and cilantro.
2. Toss the mixture with the pasta, onions, and chicken.
3. Arrange the chopped lettuce on a plate and top it with the salad mixture.
4. Top the salad with the grated carrot.

Preparation time: 10 minutes, once chicken and pasta are cooked.

Cooking time: varies according to oven temperature or microwave power level for chicken and according to directions on pasta package.

Nutrition Information per Serving:

479 calories, 39 g protein, 45 g carbohydrates, 5 g fiber,
16 g fat, 30% calories from fat, 0.74 mg vitamin B$_6$, 196 mcg folic acid,
77 mg calcium, 4 mg iron, 2 mg zinc

Salad of Many Greens (Meal)

Yield: 1 Serving

Kris uses many greens in this salad because it is the best way to ensure a wider variety of nutrients. In addition, mixing in different greens lends extra flavor to the salad. This recipe calls for garbanzo beans to supply the protein, but feel free to substitute black beans or kidney beans. I hope you find a type of mushroom you like, because mushrooms are a good source of copper, a difficult-to-get nutrient. Note that there are two versions of this dish: one as a full meal with the beans and one as a side salad without. Multiply the recipe as necessary for other family members or for another day.

> 2 cups chopped romaine lettuce
> 1 cup chopped spinach (or bagged baby spinach)
> 1 cup chopped arugula
> 1 cup canned garbanzo beans (chickpeas)
> ½ cup sliced fresh mushrooms (you can purchase them
>   this way for convenience)
> 1 tomato, chopped
>
> *Dressing:*
> 4 fresh mint leaves, chopped (about ½ tablespoon), or ½
>   teaspoon dried mint leaves
> 1 tablespoon extra-virgin olive oil
> 1 tablespoon rice wine vinegar
> 1 teaspoon honey

1. Mix together all the greens in small salad bowl. Top with the beans, mushrooms, and chopped tomato.
2. Place the mint in small bowl or large cup. Add the olive oil, vinegar, and honey and mix together with a fork. Drizzle the dressing over the salad.

Preparation time: 15 minutes

Cooking time: none

Nutrition Information per Serving:
466 calories, 16 g protein, 61 g carbohydrates, 20 g fiber,
20 g fat, 37% calories from fat, 0.32 mg vitamin B$_6$, 268 mcg folic acid,
195 mg calcium, 8 mg iron, 1.3 mg zinc

Salad of Many Greens (Side)

Yield: 1 Serving

Variety is the spice of life, and the variety of greens in this salad adds flavor and many valuable nutrients.

> 2 cups chopped romaine lettuce
> 1 cup chopped spinach (or bagged baby spinach)
> 1 cup chopped arugula
> ½ cup sliced fresh mushrooms (you can purchase them
>   this way for convenience)
> 1 tomato, chopped

> *Dressing:*
> 4 fresh mint leaves, chopped (about ½ tablespoon), or ½
>   teaspoon dried mint leaves
> 1 tablespoon extra-virgin olive oil
> 1 tablespoon rice vinegar
> 1 teaspoon honey

1. Mix together all the greens in personal salad bowl. Top them with the mushrooms and chopped tomato.
2. Chop the mint if you are using fresh (or measure out ½ teaspoon dried mint leaves) and place it in small bowl or large mug. Add the olive oil, vinegar, and honey and mix them together with a fork. Drizzle the dressing over the salad.

Preparation time: 15 minutes

Cooking time: none

Nutrition Information per Serving:
225 calories, 6 g protein, 21 g carbohydrates, 5.5 g fiber,
15 g fat, 56% calories from fat, 0.32 mg vitamin B$_6$, 268 mcg folic acid,
114 mg calcium, 4 mg iron, 1.3 mg zinc

Simple Garden Salad

Yield: 2 Servings

Although easy to make, this salad is very high in nutrients. You can make it ahead of time and just add the dressing when you're about to eat. It stores well for 2 to 3 days in the refrigerator without dressing.

> 4 cups romaine lettuce
> 1 tomato, washed and chopped
> 1 cucumber, chopped
> 2 carrots, peeled and sliced
> ¼ cup chopped fresh parsley
> ¼ cup of your favorite low-fat dressing (or 2 tablespoons
>   per serving)

1. Wash, dry, and chop the romaine lettuce; place it in a salad bowl.
2. Add the vegetables and parsley; toss the salad.
3. Split the salad between 2 salad plates and top each serving with 2 tablespoons of your favorite low-fat dressing.

Preparation time: 10 minutes

Cooking time: none

Nutrition Information per Serving:
140 calories, 5 g protein, 19 g carbohydrates, 6 g fiber,
6 g fat, 35% calories from fat, 0.28 mg vitamin B_6, 203 mcg folic acid,
94 mg calcium, 3 mg iron, 1 mg zinc

Spinach–Pear Salad

YIELD: 2 SERVINGS

A great meal in itself!

1 tablespoon extra-virgin olive oil
2 tablespoons orange juice concentrate
3 cups spinach, chopped (or bagged baby spinach)
1 fresh pear or 2 pear halves, canned in juice, sliced
1 tangerine, peeled and separated (skin segments if desired)
1 cup cooked garbanzo beans (chickpeas)
4 tablespoons walnuts, chopped
2 tablespoons fat-free croutons

1. Whisk the olive oil and juice concentrate together in a cup or small bowl; set the dressing aside.
2. Divide the spinach between two plates.
3. Arrange the pear, tangerine, and garbanzo beans on top of the spinach.
4. Drizzle the salad with the dressing and top with the walnuts and croutons.

Preparation time: 10 minutes

Cooking time: none

Nutrition Information per Serving:

385 calories, 12 g protein, 47 g carbohydrates, 11 g fiber,
19 g fat, 42% calories from fat, 0.24 mg vitamin B_6, 135 mcg folic acid,
112 mg calcium, 4 mg iron, 1 mg zinc

Tomato Salad

Yield: 1 Serving

There's nothing like the taste of oregano with tomatoes and olives. This combines spinach to give you folic acid and mozzarella cheese to give you protein. You can make this salad ahead of time and pour on the dressing when you are ready to serve. In fact, feel free to make a double batch and save one serving for another day.

1 tomato, chopped
¼ cup shredded part-skim mozzarella cheese
4 olives, chopped
¼ cup fresh oregano, chopped (or 1⅓ tablespoons dried)
2 cups spinach, chopped (or bagged baby spinach)

Dressing:
1 tablespoon extra-virgin olive oil
1 tablespoon balsamic vinegar
¼ teaspoon salt

1. Whisk all the dressing ingredients together and set the dressing aside.
2. In a salad bowl, mix the tomato, cheese, olives, oregano, and spinach; toss the salad.
3. Drizzle the salad with the dressing.

Preparation time: 10 minutes

Cooking time: none

Nutrition Information per Serving:
308 calories, 8 g protein, 16 g carbohydrates, 3 g fiber,
24 g fat, 70% calories from fat, 0.22 mg vitamin B$_6$, 135 mcg folic acid,
293 mg calcium, 2 mg iron, 1 mg zinc

Waldorf Salad

YIELD: 2 SERVINGS

Surprised to see Waldorf salad on a healthy eating menu? Don't be! Kris has made this version especially healthy, just for you and your growing baby. Don't worry, she's taken extra care to build in lots of fabulous taste. It's so enjoyable that Kris has included it occasionally as a snack.

¼ cup chopped celery
1 red apple, chopped (with peel) and tossed with a mixture
   of 2 tablespoons lemon juice and 1 tablespoon sugar to
   prevent browning
2 tablespoons chopped walnuts
2 packed tablespoons raisins
2 packed tablespoons dried cranberries (Craisins)
3 cups chopped fresh spinach

Dressing:
2 tablespoons low-fat mayonnaise
1 tablespoon lemon juice
2 teaspoons sugar

1. Combine the salad ingredients in a small mixing bowl.
2. Whisk together the dressing ingredients in a small bowl or cup.
3. Pour the dressing over the salad; toss it to mix well.
4. Place half the spinach on each of two salad plates; divide the salad between them.

Preparation time: 15 minutes

Cooking time: none

Nutrition Information per Serving:
238 calories, 3 g protein, 44 g carbohydrates, 5 g fiber,
8 g fat, 27% calories from fat, 0.21 mg vitamin B_6, 102 mcg folic acid,
72 mg calcium, 2 mg iron, 1 mg zinc

Watercress–Date Salad

Simply put: a powerhouse of taste and nutrition!

    4 cups (about 2 bunches) watercress
    12 pitted dates, halved
    ¼ cup low-fat poppyseed dressing (or 2 tablespoons per
        serving)

1. Wash the watercress, then pat it dry. Chop it (including stems) and split it between 2 salad plates.
2. Divide the halved dates between the 2 plates; drizzle each salad with 2 tablespoons poppyseed dressing (or other low-fat dressing of your choice).

Preparation time: 5 minutes

Cooking time: none

Nutrition Information per Serving:
184 calories, 3 g protein, 43 g carbohydrates, 5 g fiber,
2 g fat, 10% calories from fat, 0.18 mg vitamin B_6, 13 mcg folic acid,
98 mg calcium, 1 mg iron, 0 mg zinc

Pasta Dishes

Chicken Pasta Salad with Cilantro–Peanut Sauce

Yield: 2 Servings

This is another of Kris's personal favorites. The sauce also makes a great salad dressing.

2¼ ounces uncooked rotini pasta
6 ounces cooked chicken breast, cooled, cut into bite-size
    pieces
½ cup chopped green onion tops
2 cups chopped romaine lettuce

Sauce:
3 tablespoons smooth peanut butter
3 tablespoons light soy sauce
2 teaspoons granulated sugar
½ cup fresh coriander (cilantro) leaves

Garnish:
1 large carrot, grated

1. Cook the pasta according to the package directions. While the pasta is cooking, prepare the sauce.
2. In small food processor (or blender), combine the sauce ingredients. Process them until the cilantro is in tiny pieces. Drain the cooked pasta (do not rinse) and toss it at once with the sauce. Hot pasta absorbs the sauce much better than does cold pasta, boosting the flavor of this dish.
3. In a small mixing bowl, combine the chicken, green onion tops, and pasta and sauce; toss all to mix.
4. Serve immediately, or chill. To serve, divide the chopped lettuce between 2 dinner plates. Divide chicken–pasta mixture and place it on top of the lettuce (about 1½ cups of mixture per serving). Top each salad with half of the grated carrot.

(continued)

Preparation time: 15 minutes

*Cooking time: varies according to oven temperature
or microwave power level for chicken and according
to directions on pasta package*

Nutrition Information per Serving:
501 calories, 37 g protein, 46 g carbohydrates, 6 g fiber,
19 g fat, 34% calories from fat, 0.63 mg vitamin B_6, 222 mcg folic acid,
85 mg calcium, 5 mg iron, 3 mg zinc

Classic Spaghetti

YIELD: 2 SERVINGS

Once again, Kris has worked some magic to make an all-time favorite good for you and your baby. The mixture of ground sirloin and textured vegetable protein (TVP) is a fabulous combination—you won't even know this dish contains TVP. (Nor will your family if you don't tell them!) The TVP makes this a great source of valuable zinc.

> 2 teaspoons light olive oil
> ½ cup chopped onions
> 4 ounces lean ground sirloin
> 1½ cups canned tomato purée, no added salt
> 2 tablespoons Italian seasoning
> 1 red bell pepper, sliced
> 1 green bell pepper, sliced
> 2 ounces TVP (or substitute an additional 2 ounces lean
>   ground sirloin)
> 1½ ounces dry spinach spaghetti noodles (makes about 2
>   cups cooked)

1. Heat the olive oil and chopped onions over medium heat in a large skillet; sauté 3 minutes, or until the onions turn translucent.
2. Increase the heat to medium high and add the ground sirloin; cook until the beef is well cooked.
3. Reduce the heat to low. Add the tomato purée, Italian seasoning, bell peppers, and TVP. Cover the skillet and simmer the sauce 20 minutes.
4. While the sauce is simmering, cook the pasta according to the package directions; drain. Serve the sauce over the pasta.

Preparation time: 15 minutes

Cooking time: 20 minutes

Nutrition Information per Serving:

559 calories, 42 g protein, 71 g carbohydrates, 16 g fiber,
15 g fat, 23% calories from fat, 1.13 mg vitamin B$_6$, 153 mcg folic acid,
184 mg calcium, 8 mg iron, 13 mg zinc

Easy Cheesy Pasta Salad

Yield: 1 Serving

A fabulously easy and very nutritious lunch that travels well to work.

½ cup small shell pasta, cooked
1 cup frozen peas, thawed
2 ounces Colby cheese, shredded (or another favorite
   cheese; enough calories are allotted here for regular, not
   reduced-fat, cheese, simply because it tastes so great!)
2 tablespoons low-calorie French salad dressing

1. In a small bowl, combine the pasta, peas, and cheese.
2. Drizzle the salad with dressing and toss it.

Preparation time: 5 minutes, once pasta is cooked

Cooking time: varies according to directions on pasta package

Nutrition Information per Serving:
459 calories, 24 g protein, 45 g carbohydrates, 8 g fiber,
21 g fat, 41% calories from fat, 0.24 mg vitamin B_6, 127 mcg folic acid,
428 mg calcium, 4 mg iron, 3 mg zinc

Fresh 'n' Fruity Chicken Pasta

YIELD: 1 SERVING

Here's another great meal-in-one salad that carries to work well. The papaya makes it especially interesting and refreshing—as well as a nutrition powerhouse.

1 cup rotini pasta, cooked, drained and hot
2 tablespoons low-calorie French salad dressing
3 ounces boneless, skinless chicken breast, cooked and
   cubed
1 carrot, grated
3 cups chopped raw spinach
½ fresh papaya, sliced (approximately 5 ounces)

1. Toss the hot pasta with the salad dressing.
2. Add the chicken and grated carrots; toss the mixture.
3. Place the mixture on top of the spinach and garnish with papaya.

Preparation time: 5 minutes, once pasta and chicken are cooked

*Cooking time: varies according to oven temperature
or microwave power level for chicken and
according to directions on pasta package*

Nutrition Information per Serving:
491 calories, 37 g protein, 72 g carbohydrates, 9 g fiber,
7 g fat, 12% calories from fat, 0.87 mg vitamin B$_6$, 344 mcg folic acid,
171 mg calcium, 6 mg iron, 2 mg zinc

Legal Fettuccine Alfredo

YIELD: 2 SERVINGS

In a word: awesome. Just as important: terribly legal and very nutritious.

⅓ pound uncooked fettuccine noodles
1 tablespoon extra-virgin olive oil
1 or 2 cloves garlic, peeled and sliced thinly
¾ cup skim milk
2 tablespoons flour
2 ounces fat-free cream cheese
¼ cup shredded Parmesan cheese
½ pound frozen broccoli florets, thawed
Freshly ground black pepper to taste

1. Cook the fettuccine according to the package directions; drain.
2. While the pasta is cooking, heat the olive oil and garlic in a skillet over low heat for 5 minutes, allowing the full flavor of garlic to be released into the oil. (Be sure that the heat is very low so that the garlic doesn't brown.)
3. Meanwhile, combine the milk, flour, cream cheese, and Parmesan cheese in a blender or food processor; purée. Add the puréed mixture to the oil and garlic. Increase the heat to medium-low, and whisk the mixture continuously until it has thickened. Add the broccoli and freshly ground black pepper to taste; cover and allow broccoli to heat through (about 5 minutes). Toss the mixture with the cooked fettuccine noodles.

Preparation and cooking time: 20 minutes

Nutrition Information per Serving:
496 calories, 28 g protein, 68 g carbohydrates, 6 g fiber,
13 g fat, 23% calories from fat, 0.25 mg vitamin B_6, 62 mcg folic acid,
402 mg calcium, 1 mg iron, 1 mg zinc

Lemon-Fresh Rotini Spinach

YIELD: 2 SERVINGS

A great way to make pasta a nutrition extravaganza—and to eat more spinach.

> 3 ounces uncooked rotini pasta
> 1 tablespoon extra-virgin olive oil
> 1 clove garlic, chopped
> 1 pound spinach, chopped (or bagged baby spinach)
> 2 tablespoons fresh lemon juice
> Freshly ground black pepper to taste

1. Cook the rotini according to package directions, then drain it.
2. Return the empty pot to the burner and reduce the heat to low. Add the oil and garlic; sauté for 3 minutes.
3. Stir in the spinach and lemon juice. Cover and steam the mixture for 5 minutes. Toss it with the rotini and add the black pepper to taste.

Preparation and cooking time: 25 minutes

Nutrition Information per Serving:

278 calories, 13 g protein, 40 g carbohydrates, 8 g fiber,

9 g fat, 26% calories from fat, 0.47 mg vitamin B_6, 442 mcg folic acid,

228 mg calcium, 6 mg iron, 1 mg zinc

Peanut Papaya Pasta Salad

YIELD: 1 SERVING

You know Kris by now: always trying to get more valuable nutrients into your salads. In this dish, the papaya is high in folic acid, vitamin C, and some minerals, and the peanuts are a good source of protein, B vitamins, zinc, and copper. As a bonus, this pasta salad keeps well and survives the journey to work in tip-top shape.

¼ cup chopped fresh cilantro (coriander)
1 tablespoon extra-virgin olive oil
2 teaspoons low-sodium soy sauce
½ cup cooked rotini pasta, drained
½ cup cooked white kidney beans; also called cannellini
    beans (see "Cooking Legumes," page 218, or use canned
    beans, drained and rinsed)
2 tablespoons peanuts
1 papaya (approximately 11 ounces), peeled, seeded, and
    sliced

1. Mix the cilantro, olive oil, and soy sauce in a small bowl. Add the hot pasta and toss all.
2. Stir in the kidney beans and peanuts.
3. Fold in the papaya.
4. Chill the salad for a minimum of 1 hour; overnight is fine.

Preparation time: 10 minutes.

Cooking time: varies according to directions on pasta package

Nutrition Information per Serving:
557 calories, 15 g protein, 73 g carbohydrates, 13 g fiber,
25 g fat, 39% calories from fat, 0.15 mg vitamin B_6, 193 mcg folic acid,
134 mg calcium, 4 mg iron, 1 mg zinc

Tuna Pasta

YIELD: 4 SERVINGS

This is an old-time favorite with a healthy twist. Everyone, including the kids, will love it.

¼ cup light mayonnaise
1 tablespoon lemon juice
¼ teaspoon black pepper
3 cups cooked small pasta shells, drained and hot
½ cup chopped tomato
Two 7-ounce cans of tuna in water, drained
4 hard-boiled egg whites, chopped
1½ cups frozen green peas, thawed
8 cups spinach, chopped (or bagged baby spinach)

1. In a small bowl, whisk together the mayonnaise, lemon juice, and pepper. Toss the mixture with the hot, drained pasta.
2. Add the tomato, tuna, egg whites, and peas. Mix gently.
3. For each serving, use ¼ of this mixture over 2 cups of chopped spinach

Preparation time: 10 minutes, after pasta and eggs are cooked

Cooking time: varies according to directions on pasta package

Nutrition Information per Serving:
331 calories, 34 g protein, 39 g carbohydrates, 6 g fiber,
4 g fat, 12% calories from fat, 0.53 mg vitamin B_6, 214 mcg folic acid,
92 mg calcium, 5 mg iron, 2 mg zinc

Vegetarian Main Dishes

Cheesy Spinach Pizza

YIELD: 3 SERVINGS

Have a hankering for pizza? Try this version. It's piled high with satisfying vegetables, mozzarella cheese, and so many nutrients. If there are two of you, there's one serving left for lunch another day. It's even great cold!

Crust:
½ cup warm water
1 teaspoon dry yeast
1 teaspoon sugar
1 tablespoon olive oil
1 teaspoon salt
1⅓ cups all-purpose flour

Topping:
8-ounce can tomato sauce
2 teaspoons dried or 2 tablespoons fresh oregano
1 teaspoon garlic powder
2 teaspoons dried or 2 tablespoons fresh basil
1 medium onion, chopped
10-ounce package frozen spinach, thawed and drained
½ pound mushrooms, sliced
7.25-ounce jar roasted red peppers, drained and cut into
    1-inch pieces
6 ounces shredded 50% reduced-fat mozzarella

1. To make the crust, combine the water, yeast, and sugar; mix well. Add the olive oil and salt; mix well. Stir in the flour with a wooden spoon; beat the dough until well blended and then an additional 20 strokes. *Alternatively,* combine all the ingredients except the flour in a freestanding mixer; mix with a beater attachment until blended. Add 1 cup of the flour; mix until blended. Switch to a dough hook; add the remaining flour and beat for 2 minutes. *Alternatively,* if you have a bread machine, place all the crust ingredients in a bread machine and use the dough setting. *Alternatively,* if you don't want to make your own dough, buy frozen bread dough

(continued)

and use a 1-pound loaf. Thaw it and follow the rest of the instructions.

2. Spray a 9" pizza pan with vegetable oil spray. Place the dough in the center of the pan and pat it out over the entire pan. Let it rest for 10 minutes while you prepare the other ingredients.

3. Preheat the oven to 425° Fahrenheit. Spread the tomato sauce evenly over the dough. Sprinkle the herbs evenly over the sauce. Add the vegetables in the order given in the ingredient list. Sprinkle the mozzarella cheese evenly over the vegetables, and top everything with the feta.

4. Bake the pizza 18 to 22 minutes in the preheated oven, or until the cheese is just slightly brown and the crust is crisp.

Preparation time: 20 minutes

Cooking time: 20 minutes

Nutrition Information per Serving:

542 calories, 25 g protein, 66 g carbohydrates, 7.6 g fiber,
20 g fat, 33% calories from fat, 0.53 mg vitamin B_6, 269 mcg folic acid,
284 mg calcium, 7 mg iron, 2.5 mg zinc

Lentil Vegetable Stew

YIELD: 4 SERVINGS

This stew warms up a cool evening but tastes great anytime. This dish combines vegetables in such a way that you get all the nutrition you need in one pot. It stores and freezes well and is one of those dishes that's better as a leftover than fresh. There is something magnificent about the way parsnips and carrots combine together to create a fabulous flavor.

> 1 tablespoon extra-virgin olive oil
> 1 leek, cleaned well and sliced in ¼" slices
> 1 tablespoon vegetarian bouillon granules or paste
> Freshly ground black pepper to taste
> 1 cup uncooked lentils (you can use orange or green lentils)
> 4 large carrots (about ¾ pound), peeled and sliced thinly
> 3 small or 2 large parsnips, peeled and sliced thinly
> 1 large potato, scrubbed well and diced finely (with peel)
> 5 cups water
> ½ pound mushrooms, sliced

1. Heat the olive oil in a large nonstick skillet over low to medium heat. Add the leek, vegetarian bouillon, and black pepper, and sauté the mixture for 5 minutes, stirring it several times.
2. Add the lentils, carrots, parsnips, diced potato, and 5 cups water. Increase the heat to medium, cover the skillet, and simmer the stew 20 minutes. Stir 2 or 3 times during this cooking time. Decrease or increase heat as necessary so that the stew simmers gently.
3. Remove the skillet cover. Stir in the sliced mushrooms. Cover the skillet and simmer the stew 15 minutes more.
4. Serve the stew over cooked wild rice, brown rice, or barley. This stew stores well in the refrigerator for up to 5 days.

Preparation time: 15 minutes

*Cooking time: 35 minutes (plus variable time for
wild rice, brown rice, or barley)*

Nutrition Information per Serving:
367 calories, 16 g protein, 70 g carbohydrates, 15 g fiber,
4 g fat, 10% calories from fat, 0.49 mg vitamin B_6, 90 mcg folic acid,
114 mg calcium, 5 mg iron, 1 mg zinc

Stuffed Peppers

YIELD: 1 SERVING

Here's another recipe Kris loves to cook that's incredibly easy, especially if you've cooked up rice ahead of time and frozen it (see "Cooking Whole Grains," page 219). The roasted red peppers lend a bit of visual excitement but are gentle enough for any stomach. You can also make these ahead of time and freeze them, pulling one out for lunches as you need it. Kris often makes a batch, using several different colors of peppers. It's a gorgeous sight!

> 1 sweet red pepper (or other color as desired)
> 1 cup cooked long-grain brown rice
> ½ of 7.25-ounce jar roasted red peppers, chopped
> Olive-oil spray
> 1 cup sliced mushrooms
> ½ cup favorite jarred tomato pasta sauce

1. Preheat the oven to 350° Fahrenheit.
2. Cut the top off the sweet pepper; core the pepper and wash it; set it aside.
3. In a small bowl, mix the rice and roasted red peppers. Stuff this mixture into the cored pepper.
4. Spray a small baking dish with the olive-oil spray. Place the mushrooms in the bottom, then set the pepper on top of the sliced mushrooms. Pour the sauce over the stuffed pepper; cover the dish tightly and bake the pepper 45 minutes.

Preparation time: 10 minutes

Cooking time: 45 minutes (plus cooking time for long-grain brown rice)

Nutrition Information per Serving:
383 calories, 12 g protein, 74 g carbohydrates, 10 g fiber,
5 g fat, 13% calories from fat, 0.66 mg vitamin B_6, 53 mcg folic acid,
44 mg calcium, 4.5 mg iron, 2.3 mg zinc

Sandwiches and Wraps

Carrot–Tuna Pita

YIELD: 1 SERVING

Kris has bulked up this simple tuna sandwich with extra nutrients by adding carrots and spinach. I think you'll love the crunch that the carrots add. Be sure to look for bagged carrot matchsticks in the produce section; they're a great time saver!

    3 ounces tuna, canned in water, drained
    2 tablespoons light mayonnaise
    1 tablespoon relish
    1 carrot, shredded (or 1 cup carrot matchsticks)
    2 cups chopped spinach (or bagged baby spinach)
    1 whole-wheat pita pocket, with top cut off

1. In a small bowl, mix the tuna, mayonnaise, relish, and carrots.
2. Blend in the chopped spinach.
3. Stuff the mixture into the pita pocket.

Preparation time: 5 minutes

Cooking time: none

Nutrition Information per Serving:
403 calories, 31 g protein, 55 g carbohydrates, 9 g fiber,
9 g fat, 18% calories from fat, 0.69 mg vitamin B$_6$, 162 mcg folic acid,
98 mg calcium, 5 mg iron, 2 mg zinc

Tofu Egg Salad Sandwich

YIELD: 2 SERVINGS

Although we'd like you to use the tofu for all the nutrients it provides, you can substitute egg whites. This sandwich makes a perfect carry-to-work lunch; just make sure to put lettuce between the filling and the bread to keep the bread from getting soggy.

> 6 ounces extra-firm light tofu (or 6 cooked egg whites)
> 2 teaspoons yellow mustard (or other favorite mustard)
> 1 cup chopped celery
> 2 tablespoons light mayonnaise
> ¼ cup chopped onions
> 2 cups romaine lettuce
> 4 slices whole-wheat bread

1. In a small bowl, combine the tofu, mustard, celery, mayonnaise, and onions. Blend the mixture well with a fork.
2. Build sandwiches with the lettuce and the tofu mixture.

Preparation time: 7 minutes

Cooking time: none, unless egg whites are used

Nutrition Information per Serving:

266 calories, 14 g protein, 37 g carbohydrates, 7 g fiber,
8 g fat, 27% calories from fat, 0.39 mg vitamin B_6, 133 mcg folic acid,
144 mg calcium, 4 mg iron, 2 mg zinc

Veggie Pita

Yield: 1 Serving

The honey mustard in this creates a flavor extravaganza and combines especially well with the slightly nutty flavor of garbanzo beans.

1 carrot, grated (or 1 cup carrot matchsticks)
1 tablespoon honey mustard
½ cup canned garbanzo beans
5 cherry tomatoes, halved
1 whole-wheat pita pocket, with top cut off

1. In a small bowl, mix the carrots, mustard, beans, and tomatoes. Toss the ingredients gently to mix.
2. Stuff the mixture into a pita pocket.

Preparation time: 10 minutes

Cooking time: none

Nutrition Information per Serving:
403 calories, 15 g protein, 75 g carbohydrates, 17 g fiber,
8 g fat, 16% calories from fat, 0.46 mg vitamin B_6, 172 mcg folic acid,
134 mg calcium, 6 mg iron, 2 mg zinc

Black Bean Avocado Wrap

Wraps are the latest rage, and Kris has created some magnificent versions. She had two important factors in mind: first, she wanted them to taste so fabulous you would want to eat them over and over again. Secondly, and just as important, Kris combined the foods that would give you the widest variety of nutrients. This one is to die for!

> ½ cup cooked (see "Cooking Legumes," page 218, for
>   instructions) or canned black beans, mashed
> 3 tablespoons avocado
> 1 large whole-wheat tortilla
> *Optional:* cumin, cayenne, black pepper, and your favorite
>   salsa, to taste
> ½ cup sliced mushrooms
> ½ cup chopped tomato
> 1 cup baby corn (bought in a jar or can in the canned-
>   vegetable aisle or Asian foods section)
> 1 cup baby spinach leaves

1. Place the black beans and avocado in a small bowl and mash them with a fork. Alternatively, you can use a small food processor to purée them.
2. Spread the bean-and-avocado mixture evenly over the whole-wheat tortilla. If you desire, sprinkle with some cumin, cayenne, and black pepper and/or a layer of your favorite salsa next.
3. Sprinkle the mixture with the mushrooms, tomatoes, baby corn, and then the spinach leaves. Roll the wrap tightly and enjoy.

Preparation time: 10 minutes

Cooking time: for beans, 1½ hours

Nutrition Information per Serving:
307 calories, 16 g protein, 64 g carbohydrates, 16 g fiber,
9 g fat, 21% calories from fat, 0.35 mg vitamin B_6, 114 mcg folic acid,
91 mg calcium, 6 mg iron, 1 mg zinc

Taking Wraps to Work

Wraps are exceptionally easy to take to work. If you don't mind that the shell may become a little moist, you can construct it at home. Alternatively, take it in three parts: the tortilla shell in a plastic bag; the sauce (whatever the wet part is) in a separate container, and the veggies and greens in another container. It'll take just a moment to put it together at work.

The Wrap for the Wrap

You can be more adventurous with your wrap wrapping. Look for spinach wraps, tomato wraps, and other interesting alternatives. Wraps should have no more than about 170 calories and an upper limit of 4 grams of fat.

Chicken Wrap

YIELD: 1 SERVING

The best!

 2 tablespoons low-fat plain yogurt
 1 tablespoon favorite jarred fruit or vegetable salsa (fat free)
 1 large whole-wheat tortilla
 3 ounces skinless, boneless chicken breast, cooked and
   cubed
 ½ a 7.25-ounce jar roasted red peppers (leave pieces
   whole)
 1 cup spinach leaves

1. In a small bowl or cup, combine the yogurt and salsa. Spread the mixture over the tortilla.
2. Distribute the chicken evenly on top. Lay the roasted red pepper pieces over the chicken and then the spinach leaves on top of the peppers.
3. Roll the wrap tightly and eat it.

Preparation time: 5 minutes

*Cooking time: varies according to oven temperature
or microwave power level for chicken*

Nutrition Information per Serving:

271 calories, 33 g protein, 28 g carbohydrates, 3.5 g fiber,
4.6 g fat, 14% calories from fat, 0.67 mg vitamin B_6, 76 mcg folic acid,
122 mg calcium, 3 mg iron, 1.9 mg zinc

Five-Minute Tortilla

YIELD: 1 SERVING

A light and tasty meal in a matter of minutes.

> 1 large whole-wheat tortilla
> 1 slice cheddar-flavored soy cheese (or low-fat
>   cheddar cheese)
> ½ cup fat-free refried beans
> ¼ cup chopped sweet red bell pepper
> 1 green onion chopped, (both green and white sections)
> 1 or 2 tablespoons favorite salsa
> Olive-oil spray

1. Place the tortilla on a microwavable serving plate; spread it with the refried beans and top it with the soy cheese.
2. Microwave the tortilla on high for 1 to 2 minutes, or until it is warmed through and the cheese is melted.
3. Top it with the chopped pepper and onion and your favorite salsa.
4. Roll the tortilla and eat it.

Preparation time: 5 minutes

Cooking time: 2 minutes

Nutrition Information per Serving:
252 calories, 14 g protein, 47 g carbohydrates, 10 g fiber,
3 g fat, 9% calories from fat, 0.21 mg vitamin B_6, 38 mcg folic acid,
82 mg calcium, 3 mg iron, 1 mg zinc

Guacamole Wrap

YIELD: 1 SERVING

Yes, you read correctly. Kris has developed a form of guacamole that is actually healthy for you, especially during your days in waiting. The tiny amount of avocado adds loads of nutrients, especially copper and vitamin E, but Kris has kept the fat and calories down by blending green peas into the avocado. Kris calls for just a few spices here because many pregnant women have trouble with them, but go ahead and add whatever appeals to you: cumin, cayenne, black pepper! Kris is not a big fan of fat-free cheeses, but sometimes they are a great solution, as they are in this case. Because of the fat provided by the avocado and the olive oil, fat-free cheese becomes a necessity. It works well in this recipe and provides the extra protein you'll need in this meal.

> ¼ ripe avocado
> ½ cup frozen green peas, thawed
> 2 teaspoons olive oil
> 2 tablespoons lemon juice
> ⅛ teaspoon salt
> Pepper to taste
> Cayenne pepper to taste (if your stomach can tolerate it)
> 1 large whole-wheat tortilla
> ½ cup fat-free grated sharp cheddar cheese (equivalent to
>   2 ounces)
> 1 cup snow peas, washed and ends removed
> ¼ red pepper, thinly sliced
> ¼ yellow pepper, thinly sliced

1. Mash the avocado and thawed peas with a fork; blend in the olive oil, lemon juice, salt, and pepper to taste (and other spices if you are using them). Alternatively, place all of these ingredients in a small food processor and purée.
2. Spread the avocado mixture over the tortilla evenly. Top it with cheese.

(continued)

3. Arrange the snow peas and pepper slices evenly over the tortilla. Roll it tightly.

Preparation time: 10 minutes

Cooking time: none

Nutrition Information per Serving:
440 calories, 31 g protein, 49 g carbohydrates, 11.6 g fiber,
17.6 g fat, 33% calories from fat, 0.57 mg vitamin B_6, 135 mcg folic acid,
572 mg calcium, 4.2 mg iron, 4.2 mg zinc

Hummus Wrap

Yield: 1 Serving

Hummus is a fabulous nutrition secret from the Middle East. Its gentle flavor is complemented by a host of many nutrients you need now (and every day!). Roasted pumpkin seeds blend well with the flavor of hummus and add many of the minerals you and your baby need every day. You'll love the combination of flavors and textures in this fun wrap.

> 1 large whole-wheat tortilla
> ½ cup hummus (you can buy it in the deli or health-food
>   store or make your own; see recipe on page 342)
> 1 tablespoon roasted pumpkin seeds
> ¼ sweet red bell pepper, in slices
> ¼ sweet yellow bell pepper, in slices
> 1 cup baby spinach leaves

1. Spread the hummus over the tortilla.
2. Sprinkle on pumpkin seeds and gently push them into the hummus (so they don't fall out while you are eating the wrap).
3. Arrange the pepper slices and then the spinach leaves; roll the tortilla tightly.

Preparation time: 10 minutes

Cooking time: none

Nutrition Information per Serving:
325 calories, 15 g protein, 45 g carbohydrates, 11 g fiber,
13 g fat, 33% calories from fat, 0.53 mg vitamin B_6, 189 mcg folic acid,
97 mg calcium, 5.07 mg iron, 3.5 mg zinc

Roasted Red Pepper and Beef Wraps

YIELD: 2 SERVINGS

Kris has designed this recipe for one of those nights when you are short on time or energy—or both. To make it really fast, buy beef already cut for stir-frying.

> 2 teaspoons light olive oil
> ⅓ cup chopped red onion
> 2 teaspoons very low sodium beef bouillon granules
> ½ pound very lean beef, sliced thinly for stir-fry (all fat removed)
> 2 cups frozen broccoli florets
> 7.5-ounce jar roasted red peppers (packed in water), chopped
> Freshly ground black pepper to taste
> 2 large whole-wheat tortillas

1. Heat the oil over medium heat with the onion and beef bouillon granules; sauté until the onion is translucent.
2. Increase the heat to medium high; add the beef, broccoli, and chopped peppers. Stir-fry the mixture until the beef is cooked. Add freshly ground black pepper to taste.
3. Place half of the mixture on each tortilla; roll the tortillas and eat.

Preparation time: 10 minutes

Cooking time: 10 minutes

Nutrition Information per Serving:
370 calories, 31 g protein, 43 g carbohydrates, 6 g fiber,
11 g fat, 25% calories from fat, 0.4 mg vitamin B_6, 26 mcg folic acid,
57 mg calcium, 5 mg iron, 5 mg zinc

Sweet Walnut Wrap

YIELD: 1 SERVING

When Kris was developing these recipes, this was her favorite wrap! It's so incredibly easy yet bursting with nutrients. Walnut oil is one secret, as is the sweet melody created by the soybeans and the honey. Make your life easy by looking for carrot matchsticks in the produce section and for mesclun greens bagged and washed. Green soybeans, also called edamame beans, can usually be found in the frozen-vegetable section of your supermarket; you can find them fresh at some specialty food stores.

¼ cup plain low-fat yogurt
1 teaspoon walnut oil
2 teaspoons honey
1 large whole-wheat tortilla
⅔ cup cooked green soybeans, cooked and cooled (see
   "Cooking Legumes," page 218, regarding cooking fresh
   soybeans)
1 cup grated carrot (or carrot matchsticks bought in a bag
   in the produce section)
1 cup mesclun greens

1. In a small bowl, whisk together the yogurt, walnut oil, and honey. Spread the mixture evenly over a whole-wheat tortilla.
2. Sprinkle the soybeans and carrots evenly over tortilla. Add mesclun greens and roll the tortilla tightly.

Preparation time: 10 minutes

*Cooking time: varies according to the use of fresh
versus frozen soybeans*

Nutrition Information per Serving:
418 calories, 23 g protein, 61 g carbohydrates, 11 g fiber,
14 g fat, 27% calories from fat, 0.39 mg vitamin B_6, 222 mcg folic acid,
356 mg calcium, 5 mg iron, 3 mg zinc

Beef, Fish, Pork, and Poultry

Crock-Pot Flank Steak and Mushrooms

Using a Crock-Pot makes this meal so easy. Also, Kris uses frozen peas instead of fresh ones, which also makes this easy and accessible. Buy the mushrooms already sliced so you have very little preparation work. If you don't have a Crock-Pot, Kris included directions for making this in a conventional oven. She's used pearl barley instead of rice in this recipe because it has more of the copper and zinc that you and your baby need. Also, Kris thinks you'll enjoy its creamy, rich texture with this stewlike dreamy rich meal.

> 1 pound lean flank steak
> 1 can reduced-sodium cream of mushroom soup
> 2 tablespoons balsamic vinegar
> 1 pound mushrooms, sliced
> 1 cup frozen peas
> 2 cups cooked pearl barley (see "Cooking Whole Grains,"
>   page 219)

1. Cut the flank steak into 4 pieces and place them in a Crock-Pot.
2. Add the soup and balsamic vinegar.
3. Cook the mixture for 3 to 12 hours on high.*
4. About 1 hour before serving, add the sliced mushrooms and frozen peas.
5. At the end of the cooking time, slice the meat, reserving half for sandwiches another day.
6. Split the remaining meat, mushrooms, and peas (and sauce). Serve the dish over cooked barley.

Preparation time: 5 minutes

Cooking time: 3 hours

Nutrition Information per Serving:
503 calories, 36 g protein, 55 g carbohydrates, 11 g fiber,
17 g fat, 30% calories from fat, 0.69 mg vitamin B_6, 106 mcg folic acid,
74 mg calcium, 8 mg iron, 7 mg zinc

---

*If you don't have a Crock-Pot, place the meat, soup, and balsamic vinegar in a heavy casserole dish, cover it, and bake it at 300° Fahrenheit for 2 hours. Uncover the dish, add the mushrooms and peas; cover and cook 20 minutes longer.

The Best Hamburger

YIELD: 2 SERVINGS

Satisfy the craving for hearty beef with this fabulously interesting burger. It's so nutritionally complete, it really is a meal in a bun.

> 3 tablespoons balsamic vinegar
> 2 tablespoons olive oil
> 1 tablespoon chopped fresh basil
> 1 clove garlic, crushed
> ¼ teaspoon ground black pepper
> 2 teaspoons sugar
> 2 large portobello mushroom caps, washed and patted dry
> 6 ounces very lean ground sirloin
> Salt and pepper to taste
> 2 whole-grain hamburger buns
> 2 thick tomato slices
> 2 large leaves romaine lettuce
> 4 teaspoons nonfat blue cheese dressing

1. In a shallow container, mix the balsamic vinegar, olive oil, basil, garlic, ¼ teaspoon black pepper, and sugar. Place the mushroom caps in, top side down. Spoon the marinade into the bottom of the caps. Cover and marinate them for 1 hour at room temperature or overnight in the refrigerator.
2. Divide the ground sirloin into 2 patties, adding salt and pepper as desired.
3. Grill the sirloin patties for 5 minutes on one side, then flip them. After flipping the patties, add the mushroom caps to the grill (or broiler pan), top side up (discard marinade). Grill both an additional 5 minutes, or until the mushrooms are slightly brown and the patties are no longer pink in the middle.
4. Build the portobello burger: Place 1 teaspoon blue cheese dressing on the bottom of the bun; add a sirloin patty, then a tomato slice and a mushroom cap; place 1 teaspoon blue cheese dressing on top of the mushroom; add the bun top.

Preparation time: 10 minutes

Cooking time: 10 minutes

Nutrition Information per Serving:

500 calories, 22 g protein, 36 g carbohydrates, 4 g fiber,
31 g fat, 55% calories from fat, 0.30 mg vitamin B_6, 65 mcg folic acid,
74 mg calcium, 4 mg iron, 4 mg zinc

Ginger-Seared Chilean Sea Bass

YIELD: 2 SERVINGS

If you haven't tried sea bass, treat yourself! This fish tastes incredibly rich but is actually quite lean. Its flavors mingle well with the sesame, ginger, and cilantro that top off this gourmet meal. Use this for guests or for yourself when you want something special. When you prepare this meal, you'll think you're using way too much Swiss chard, simply because this amount makes such a mound. Don't worry, it cooks down to about a fifth of the original size. Be sure and try it, as Swiss chard is loaded with nutrients—and taste!

> 1 teaspoon dark sesame oil
> ¼ cup finely chopped fresh ginger (or bottled chopped ginger)
> ½ pound Chilean sea bass (or salmon or cod)
> 1 pound red Swiss chard, julienned
> ½ cup chopped green onions
> ½ cup fresh cilantro (coriander), chopped
> 3 tablespoons reduced-sodium soy sauce
> ½ cup grated carrot

1. Heat the sesame oil and ginger in large nonstick skillet over medium-high heat. Add the sea bass, searing each side for 2 minutes.
2. Reduce the heat to medium. Remove the sea bass from the skillet. Place the Swiss chard in the bottom of the skillet. Top with the sea bass, then the green onions, cilantro, and soy sauce.
3. Cover the skillet tightly and simmer the chard and sea bass for 15 to 20 minutes, or until the fish flakes. The Swiss chard will quickly create more cooking liquid. Baste the mixture twice during cooking time with the cooking juices.
4. Divide the vegetables and fish between 2 plates. Garnish each with ¼ cup grated carrot.

Preparation time: 15 minutes

Cooking time: 20 minutes

Nutrition Information per Serving:
247 calories, 33 g protein, 17 g carbohydrates, 7 g fiber,
6 g fat, 21% calories from fat, 0.88 mg vitamin B_6, 70 mcg folic acid,
170 mg calcium, 6 mg iron, 2 mg zinc

Roasted Red Pepper and Trout Roll-Ups

Yield: 2 Servings

Kris loves this incredibly easy yet fancy meal. Plan it for an especially romantic evening or for guests.

>2 trout fillets (about 8 ounces each, with skin) or flounder
>   fillets
>2 teaspoons plus 2 tablespoons cooking sherry wine
>6 large fresh basil leaves
>7.25-ounce jar roasted red peppers (not in oil)
>½ tablespoon light olive oil
>¼ pound fresh mushrooms, chopped
>1 teaspoon 33%-reduced-sodium chicken bouillon granules
>2 teaspoons very low sodium chicken bouillon granules
>1 cup water
>2 cups cooked wild rice (or brown or white rice)

1. Place each trout fillet on a piece of aluminum foil about twice the size of the fillet.
2. Rub 1 teaspoon of sherry evenly over the surface of each fillet.
3. Place 3 basil leaves on each fillet, topping each with ¼ of the roasted red peppers from the jar.
4. Roll each fillet, starting at the smaller end. Then wrap foil around the rolled fillet. Set it aside.
5. Heat the oil in a large skillet over medium-high heat. Add the mushrooms, bouillon, remaining sherry, and water. Place the foil-wrapped fillets on top of the mushrooms. Cover the skillet tightly and cook the fillets 20 minutes. Check the water occasionally, adding more if it cooks away.
6. Unwrap the fillets and serve over the mushrooms and wild rice.

Preparation time: 10 minutes

Cooking time: 20 minutes (plus time for cooking rice)

Nutrition Information per Serving:
593 calories, 61 g protein, 46 g carbohydrates, 4 g fiber,
16 g fat, 25% calories from fat, 1.06 mg vitamin B_6, 99 mcg folic acid,
216 mg calcium, 3 mg iron, 4 mg zinc

Salmon in a Tarragon–Orange Cream Sauce

YIELD: 2 SERVINGS

Although salmon is always fabulous grilled alone, it is also complemented so well by other flavors. Try this, one of Kris's favorite fish recipes, for a special occasion.

Marinade:
½ cup orange juice
Zest from 1 orange
1 thinly sliced orange (discard the ends)
¼ cup fresh tarragon leaves, chopped finely
Freshly ground black pepper to taste
2 teaspoons maple syrup

Two 5-ounce salmon fillets

Sauce:
½ tablespoon nonfat sour cream
1 tablespoon Madeira wine (or white wine or white wine
　　vinegar)
2 tablespoons orange juice, into which you have blended
　　2 teaspoons cornstarch

1. To marinate the fish, combine the orange juice, orange zest, tarragon leaves, black pepper, and maple syrup in a shallow container. Add the salmon, flesh side down. Place the orange slices on top. Cover the dish tightly and marinate at least 2 hours, up to a maximum of 12 hours.
2. To cook, transfer the contents of the marinating container to a glass baking dish (fish flesh side down, with the orange slices and marinade); cover the dish with foil and bake the fish at 350° Fahrenheit for 30 minutes.
3. Remove the liquid from the dish; pour it into a small saucepan and place it on a burner over medium-low heat. Cover the fish to keep it warm. Squeeze the extra juice from the orange slices into the saucepan. Whisk in the sour cream, wine, and orange juice–cornstarch mixture; stir until the sauce thickens.
4. Remove the skin from the salmon and transfer the fish to serving plates. Divide the sauce between the 2 fish servings.

Preparation time: 10 minutes, plus at least 2 hours' marinating time

Cooking time: 35 minutes

Nutrition Information per Serving:

452 calories, 41 g protein, 31 g carbohydrates, 2 g fiber,
16 g fat, 32% calories from fat, 0.38 mg vitamin B$_6$, 50 mcg folic acid,
75 mg calcium, 1 mg iron, 1 mg zinc

Sweet-and-Sour Salmon Steaks

YIELD: 2 SERVINGS

The salmon marries beautifully with the sweet and sour flavors of the other ingredients to create a delicious meal in double-quick time.

1 tablespoon light olive oil
½ cup chopped red onion
Two 4-ounce salmon steaks
¼ teaspoon salt
1 teaspoon freshly ground black pepper
1 cup unsweetened pineapple juice
2 tablespoons vinegar
½ each green, yellow, and red sweet bell peppers, chopped
½ cup orange juice, into which you have mixed 1 tablespoon cornstarch and 1 tablespoon granulated sugar
1 cup cooked brown rice

1. Heat the light olive oil and chopped red onion in large nonstick skillet, sautéeing over medium heat until the onion has wilted.
2. Increase the heat to high; add the fish, salt, and pepper. Sear each side 2 minutes.
3. Reduce the heat to medium-low; add the pineapple juice, vinegar, and sweet peppers. Simmer the mixture 10 minutes covered, or until the salmon flakes.
4. Uncover the skillet and remove the fish. Blend in orange juice–cornstarch–sugar mixture and stir until the liquid is thickened.
5. Top each steak with half of the vegetable-and-sauce mixture and serve with brown rice.

Preparation time: 10 minutes

Cooking time: 15 minutes (plus cooking time for brown rice)

Nutrition Information per Serving:
537 calories, 44 g protein, 67 g carbohydrates, 4 g fiber,
10 g fat, 17% calories from fat, 1.9 mg vitamin B_6, 86 mcg folic acid,
180 mg calcium, 4 mg iron, 2 mg zinc

Tuna Melt

YIELD: 2 SERVINGS

Did you know that canned tuna is just as nutritious as fresh? It has just as much of those great omega-3 fatty acids and of vitamin B$_6$; though it can be a little higher in sodium, you can buy the sodium-reduced version if you're concerned. It's great to have a few cans on hand to mix up an easy dinner such as this Tuna Melt. If you haven't tried soy cheese, please do. Many brands come in several flavors. Kris likes to use it in recipes because it is so much lower in fat and so much higher in the nutrients that you and your growing baby are looking for.

> 6-ounce can tuna packed in water, drained
> 1 tbsp. low-fat Miracle Whip or mayonnaise
> Ground black pepper to taste
> 2 stalks celery, chopped
> 1 carrot, grated
> 1 small onion, minced
> 2 whole-wheat English muffins
> 4 slices low-fat soy cheddar cheese (or substitute regular, low-fat cheese)

1. Mix the tuna, Miracle Whip, pepper, celery, carrot, and onion in a small mixing bowl.
2. Open the English muffins; divide the tuna mixture evenly between the 4 halves. Top with the cheese.
3. Place the sandwiches under the broiler (or in a toaster oven) and broil them until the cheese starts to bubble and turn golden (about 2 to 3 minutes).

Preparation time: 5 minutes

Cooking time: 10 minutes

Nutrition Information per Serving:
302 calories, 29 g protein, 37 g carbohydrates, 7 g fiber,
5 g fat, 14% calories from fat, 0.56 mg vitamin B$_6$, 58 mcg folic acid,
238 mg calcium, 3 mg iron, 2 mg zinc

Scalloped Potatoes

YIELD: 2 SERVINGS
(double the recipe if you want leftovers)

Who doesn't love creamy, rich scalloped potatoes? Potatoes are such a great food, especially when you leave the peel on to get extra fiber and nutrients. This stores well in the refrigerator and carries well to work.

½ pound red-skin potatoes, with peel
¼ pound very lean ham (okay to use very lean luncheon
    meat) or lean Canadian bacon, chopped or diced
1½ cups skim milk
2 tablespoons all-purpose flour
1 tablespoon olive oil
½ cup chopped onions
2 ounces reduced-fat cheddar cheese

1. Preheat the oven to 350° Fahrenheit.
2. Scrub the potatoes and slice them thinly (with the peel left on).
3. Spray a large, shallow casserole dish with vegetable oil and add all the ingredients except the cheese. Stir them well.
4. Bake the mixture for 1 to 1½ hours, or until all liquid has evaporated and the mixture has thickened; stir the mixture twice during baking.
5. Sprinkle the cheese on top and bake the potatoes 10 minutes more or until the cheese bubbles.

Preparation time: 15 minutes

Cooking time: 70 to 100 minutes

Nutrition Information per Serving:
359 calories, 25 g protein, 41 g carbohydrates, 3 g fiber,
9 g fat, 25% calories from fat, 0.43 mg vitamin B_6, 47 mcg folic acid,
361 mg calcium, 2 mg iron, 2 mg zinc

Chicken Pot Pie Without the Pie

YIELD: 2 SERVINGS

We all love those frozen chicken pot pies—but they are generally loaded with fat. One of the reasons chicken pot pies are so high in fat is that pie crusts are by nature high in fat. That's why Kris created this version. It's so tasty, you won't even miss the crust.

> 3 tablespoons all-purpose flour
> 4 teaspoons 33%-reduced-sodium chicken bouillon
>   granules
> ½ pound skinless, boneless chicken, roasted, and cubed
> 2 tablespoons light olive oil
> ½ teaspoon chopped garlic (about 1 or 2 cloves)
> 2 carrots, peeled and sliced
> ½ pound potatoes, scrubbed and diced (with skin)
> 1 cup frozen peas

1. Mix the flour and bouillon in a small bowl; toss the chicken in this mixture and set it aside.
2. Heat the olive oil in a skillet with garlic over low heat; sauté briefly. Increase the heat to medium high; add the chicken and stir-fry until the chicken is browned.
3. Add ½ cup water, carrots, and potatoes; cover the skillet and simmer the mixture for 20 minutes. Add the frozen peas, cover the skillet, and simmer the mixture for 10 minutes more.
4. Serve.

Preparation time: 10 minutes

Cooking time: 30 minutes (plus time for cooking chicken)

Nutrition Information per Serving:
546 calories, 44 g protein, 50 g carbohydrates, 8 g fiber,
18 g fat, 30% calories from fat, 1.24 mg vitamin B_6, 75 mcg folic acid,
66 mg calcium, 4 mg iron, 3 mg zinc

Creamy Chicken Noodle Casserole

YIELD: 4 SERVINGS

Everyone loves a chicken noodle casserole, and it's especially great for those nights when you have a queasy stomach. Kris has put vegetables in here to make a complete meal—frozen ones at that so that you don't have to do any prep work. If you are low on energy or short on time, look for precooked chicken in the grocery meat case. The cornflakes on the top lend an interesting crunch. Another reason to use cornflakes on the top: They're fortified with lots of vitamins and minerals you and your baby are looking for.

> 1 can condensed cream of chicken soup
> 3 tablespoons all-purpose flour
> 1 cup skim milk
> ¼ teaspoon black pepper
> ½ cup chopped onions
> 4 cups frozen peas and carrots
> ¾ pound skinless, boneless chicken breast, cooked and cubed
> 2 tablespoons very low sodium chicken bouillon granules
> 3 cups cooked egg noodles
> 1 cup cornflakes cereal
> Olive-oil spray

1. Preheat the oven to 350° Fahrenheit.
2. In a medium casserole dish, mix the soup, flour, and skim milk until they are well blended.
3. Stir in the pepper, onions, peas, carrots, and cooked chicken.
4. Fold in the cooked egg noodles.
5. Bake the casserole, uncovered, at 350° Fahrenheit for 30 minutes.
6. Remove it from the oven, sprinkle cornflakes over the top, and spray it with the olive-oil spray.
7. Return the casserole to the oven, uncovered, and bake it an additional 10 minutes.

Preparation time: 15 minutes

Cooking time: 40 minutes (plus cooking time for chicken)

Nutrition Information per Serving:

539 calories, 42 g protein, 70 g carbohydrates, 7 g fiber,
10 g fat, 17% calories from fat, 0.87 mg vitamin B_6, 164 mcg folic acid,
166 mg calcium, 7 mg iron, 3 mg zinc

Roasted Chicken and Veggies

YIELD: 2 SERVINGS
(with lots of leftover chicken)

Another great meal-in-one with a few different vegetables, to make sure you get a blend of different nutrients. If you haven't tried Brussels sprouts, this is a wonderfully mild way to do so. They are a great source of folic acid and fiber.

3- to 5-pound roasting chicken
Olive-oil spray
1 bunch (about ¼ cup) fresh rosemary (or 1 tablespoon
    dried rosemary)
1 tablespoon instant chicken bouillon granules
1 pound small red potatoes, scrubbed, with skin on
4 large carrots, peeled, ends removed
½ pound Brussels sprouts, cleaned
½ cup balsamic vinegar, divided into 2 portions
½ teaspoon salt
½ teaspoon black pepper
½ teaspoon garlic powder

1. Preheat the oven to 400° Fahrenheit.
2. Wash the chicken, inside and out. Remove any fat pads.
3. Spray a roasting pan lightly with the olive-oil spray. Place the whole chicken in, breast up.
4. Place the fresh rosemary and bouillon granules in the chicken cavity.
5. Arrange the vegetables around the chicken. Pour ¼ cup balsamic vinegar over the top. Sprinkle the chicken with salt, pepper, and garlic powder.
6. Bake it for 20 minutes, uncovered.
7. Remove it from the oven and pour off all drippings.
8. Pour ¼ cup more balsamic vinegar over the top of the chicken.
9. Cover it tightly and reduce the oven temperature to 325° Fahrenheit and bake the chicken for 1½ hours.

(continued)

10. Remove the chicken from the oven and serve it with the vege-tables. A serving is 4 ounces of chicken meat (no skin, no bones) and half of the carrots, half of the Brussels sprouts, and half of the potatoes.

Preparation time: 5 minutes

Cooking time: 2 hours

Nutrition Information per Serving:

504 calories, 46 g protein, 68 g carbohydrates, 14 g fiber,

5 g fat, 9% calories from fat, 1.15 mg vitamin B_6, 98 mcg folic acid,

135 mg calcium, 6 mg iron, 3 mg zinc

Ten-Minute Chicken Stir-Fry

YIELD: 2 SERVINGS

Using frozen veggies and already cooked chicken makes this a snap. You can change this recipe around, using different kinds of frozen stir-fry blends to make totally different meals. If the garlic or onions bother you, just leave them out.

1 tablespoon light olive oil
½ cup chopped onions
2 cloves garlic, chopped
1 tablespoon very low sodium chicken bouillon granules
1 pound bag of vegetable stir-fry, such as Broccoli Stir-Fry
    by Fresh Like brand; avoid those with sauces
2 tablespoons of favorite stir-fry sauce
8 ounces of leftover precooked chicken or "shortcut"
    cooked chicken, your favorite flavor
½ 10-ounce bag of carrot matchsticks (available in produce
    department at your grocery store)

1. Heat the oil in a nonstick pan over medium-high heat with the onions, garlic, chicken bouillon granules, and bag of frozen vegetables. Sauté them for 5 minutes.
2. Add the stir-fry sauce, chicken, and carrot matchsticks. Sauté the ingredients briefly until all are heated through. The carrot matchsticks should still be crisp, lending a great texture.

Preparation time: 3 minutes

Cooking time: 7 minutes

Nutrition Information per Serving:
465 calories, 42 g protein, 34 g carbohydrates, 8 g fiber,
16 g fat, 32% calories from fat, 0.87 mg vitamin B_6, 22 mcg folic acid,
113 mg calcium, 3 mg iron, 1 mg zinc

Vegetables and Side Dishes

Cream Cheese Whipped Potatoes and Gravy

YIELD: 4 SERVINGS
(makes great leftovers!)

An even tastier version of the ultimate comfort food!

Whipped Potatoes:
1 pound potatoes
⅓ cup nonfat milk
2 tablespoons low-fat cream cheese
2 tablespoons nonfat sour cream
½ teaspoon salt
Black pepper to taste

1. Peel the potatoes; cut them into small chunks and place them in a saucepan. Cover them with water; bring the water to a boil, then simmer the potatoes until fork-tender, about 20 to 30 minutes.
2. Drain them and return them to the pot, reducing the heat to low. Add the remainder of the ingredients and heat through (potatoes mash better when the other ingredients are warm). *Alternatively:* Cook the potatoes per step 1 ahead of time, then drain, cover, and refrigerate them in a microwave-safe container. Just before serving, add the remainder of ingredients and microwave them until hot, about 6 minutes total—stopping to stir once at 3 minutes. Whip them per step 3.
3. Mash the potato mixture until smooth, using a hand mixer or an electric mixer.

Potato preparation time: 10 minutes

Potato cooking time: 30 minutes

Nutrition Information per Serving of cream cheese whipped potatoes:
130 calories, 4 g protein, 26 g carbohydrates, 2 g fiber,
1 g fat, 10% calories from fat, 0.32 mg vitamin B$_6$, 12 mcg folic acid,
51 mg calcium, 1 mg iron, 0 mg zinc

(continued)

Gravy:
1 cup water
2 teaspoons regular chicken bouillon granules
1 tablespoon very low sodium chicken bouillon granules
2 tablespoons cornstarch stirred into ¼ cup water
Black pepper to taste

1. Heat the water with the bouillon granules over high heat.
2. When the liquid comes to a boil, whisk in the cornstarch paste, stirring constantly.
3. Remove the mixture from heat when it thickens appropriately. Stir in the pepper.

Gravy preparation and cooking time: 10 minutes

Nutrition Information per Serving of gravy:
25 calories, 0 g protein, 6 g carbohydrates, 0 g fiber,
0 g fat, 0% calories from fat, 0 mg vitamin B_6, 0 mcg folic acid,
0 mg calcium, 0 mg iron, 0.44 mg zinc

Herb and Apple Stuffing

YIELD: 4 SERVINGS

Mouthwatering as a stuffing for turkey or chicken, this is also great on its own.

½ large yellow onion, chopped
2 red apples (not Delicious; they just don't cook well),
    chopped into bite-size squares (with skin) and tossed
    with 1 or 2 tablespoons lemon juice to prevent browning
¾ cup chopped celery
½ cup chopped fresh sage
½ pound whole-grain bread (such as a 12-grain bread), cut
    into chunks (preferably, cut bread into chunks and allow
    it to stand uncovered overnight to dry out slightly)
1 teaspoon poultry seasoning
½ to 1 teaspoon ground black pepper
2 teaspoons regular chicken bouillon granules
2 tablespoons very low sodium chicken bouillon granules
1½ cups hot water

1. Combine the onion, apples, celery, sage, bread, poultry seasoning, and black pepper in a large mixing bowl.
2. Mix together the regular and very low sodium bouillon granules with hot water until the bouillon is well dissolved; pour it over the dressing mixture. Mix well until the bread is evenly wet.
3. Stuff the mixture into a turkey, or bake it separately in a bowl. This mixture flavors your turkey beautifully, so don't hesitate to stuff your bird. If you do stuff it, wash the interior of the turkey and dry it with a paper towel. Stuff it just before baking and then bake immediately. Follow your favorite cookbook's directions for baking a stuffed turkey, which requires extra baking time. Alternatively, bake the stuffing separately uncovered at 350° Fahrenheit for 1 hour.

Preparation time: 15 minutes

Cooking time: 1 hour (excluding turkey)

Nutrition Information per Serving:
216 calories, 6 g protein, 44 g carbohydrates, 6 g fiber,
3 g fat, 11% calories from fat, 0.26 mg vitamin B_6, 57 mcg folic acid,
98 mg calcium, 2 mg iron, 1 mg zinc

Sweet-Potato Fries

YIELD: 2 SERVINGS

Bet you can't eat just one!

> 1 pound sweet potatoes
> 1 tablespoon extra-virgin olive oil
> 1 teaspoon brown sugar
> ¼ teaspoon salt

1. Preheat the oven to 375° Fahrenheit.
2. Peel the sweet potatoes and slice them thinly. In a small bowl or cup, mix the olive oil with the brown sugar and salt. Pour the mixture in the center of a cookie sheet that has a lip.
3. Dip each side of the sweet-potato slices in the sauce and spread them evenly over the cookie sheet.
4. Bake the fries 20 minutes, turning them after 10 minutes.

Preparation time: 10 minutes

Cooking time: 20 minutes

Nutrition Information per Serving:

305 calories, 4 g protein, 57 g carbohydrates, 7 g fiber,
7 g fat, 21% calories from fat, 0.55 mg vitamin B_6, 51 mcg folic acid,
66 mg calcium, 1 mg iron, 1 mg zinc

Sweet Potatoes in an Orange–Brown Sugar Glaze

Yield: 2 Servings

Sweet potatoes aren't just for Thanksgiving. Try this for a delicious, sweet vegetable side dish.

>1 pound sweet potatoes
>
>*Sauce:*
>1 tablespoon light olive oil
>1 tablespoon brown sugar
>1 teaspoon cinnamon
>2 tablespoons orange juice

1. Bake the sweet potatoes (with the skin on) until fork-tender in a conventional oven at 350° Fahrenheit, for about 30 to 40 minutes, depending on their size. For microwave baking, pierce the potatoes several times with fork, wrap them in wax paper, and microwave them on high for 3 minutes. Turn them and then microwave them for an additional 3 minutes, or until fork-tender.
2. Peel the potatoes when they are cool to the touch. Cut into 1"-thick slices.
3. Heat the oil in a nonstick pan over low heat. Add the brown sugar and cinnamon and stir the mixture until a thick sauce forms. Stir in the orange juice, making sure the heat is low so that the orange juice doesn't burn.
4. Add the sweet-potato slices, coating them with the sauce. Cover the pan and allow the sweet potatoes to heat through, about 10 minutes.

Preparation time: 10 minutes

Cooking time: 40 minutes

Nutrition Information per Serving:
316 calories, 4 g protein, 63 g carbohydrates, 7 g fiber,
6 g fat, 16% calories from fat, 0.56 mg vitamin B_6, 78 mcg folic acid,
71 mg calcium, 1 mg iron, 1 mg zinc

Desserts, Smoothies, Shakes, and Snacks

DESSERTS

SMOOTHIES AND SHAKES

SNACKS

Banana Split

YIELD: 1 SERVING

For those days when you simply must have a banana split!

½ cup of your favorite ice cream (not low fat)
2 tablespoons fat-free chocolate syrup
1 cup sliced fresh strawberries
1 banana, sliced
2 tablespoons fat-free frozen whipped topping
1 tablespoon sliced almonds or walnuts

1. Mix the strawberries and banana in a cereal bowl.
2. Top them with ½ cup of your favorite rich ice cream.
3. Drizzle everything with chocolate syrup, top with whipped topping, and sprinkle with almonds or walnuts.

Preparation time: 5 minutes

Cooking time: none

Nutrition Information per Serving:
391 calories, 6 g protein, 71 g carbohydrates, 8 g fiber,
12 g fat, 25% calories from fat, 0.82 mg vitamin B$_6$, 59 mcg folic acid,
134 mg calcium, 1 mg iron, 1 mg zinc

Chocolate Fudge Brownies

YIELD: 12 SERVINGS

Here's a brownie recipe packed with an incredibly healthy surprise! Although puréed black beans are an unusual ingredient in fudge brownies, they give a great texture and moistness (plus extra fiber) without adding any extra fat. Try it—you'll love it! (And Kris promises you won't even taste the beans.)

> 1 cup granulated sugar
> ½ cup white flour
> ¼ cup light olive oil
> ½ cup puréed cooked black beans (see "Cooking
>   Legumes," page 218, for cooking your own beans, or buy
>   canned black beans and drain, rinse, and purée them in
>   a food processor)
> ½ cup liquid egg substitute or 4 egg whites
> 2 squares unsweetened baking chocolate, melted
> 2 tablespoons pure vanilla extract
> Olive-oil spray
> 1 tablespoon sifted powdered sugar

1. Preheat the oven to 350° Fahrenheit.
2. Mix together the sugar and flour in a large mixing bowl.
3. Whisk in the oil, puréed black beans, egg substitute (or egg whites), melted chocolate, and vanilla extract.
4. Spray a 9" × 9" pan with the olive-oil spray. Scrape the batter into the pan. Bake the brownies for approximately 25 minutes. They will be slightly jiggly in the middle.
5. Sprinkle them with the powdered sugar.
6. Cut the brownies into 12 squares.

Preparation time: 15 minutes

Cooking time: 25 minutes

Nutrition Information per Serving:
171 calories, 3 g protein, 24 g carbohydrates, 1 g fiber,
8 g fat, 37% calories from fat, 0.01 mg vitamin B$_6$, 10 mcg folic acid,
14 mg calcium, 1 mg iron, 0 mg zinc

Orange Cream Fruit Tarts

Yield: 16 Servings

Kris's family loves sugar cookies, so she worked hard to develop a recipe that wasn't so high in saturated fat. Then she decided to make the tarts even healthier by loading them up with fruit. These tarts disappear in about 1 hour in her house! They do take a little more time and effort to make than the other desserts in this section, but they're great for a romantic dinner or if you're entertaining.

Crust:
1 cup margarine
3 ounces fat-free cream cheese
1 cup granulated sugar
½ teaspoon salt
1 teaspoon almond extract
2 egg whites
2 tablespoons freshly squeezed orange juice
   (or bottled juice)
1 tablespoon plus 1 teaspoon orange zest
2¼ cups flour
Olive-oil spray

Sauce/Frosting:
1 cup yogurt cheese (made from 1 pint fat-free
   vanilla yogurt)
¼ cup powdered sugar
2 tablespoons canola-based tub margarine
2 teaspoons orange zest
1 teaspoon orange juice

Fruit:
2 kiwis, sliced, each slice quartered
1 can mandarin oranges, drained and patted dry
1 cup sliced strawberries
1 banana, sliced and tossed with orange juice, then drained

(continued)

1. Make the yogurt cheese the night before you'll be making the tarts: Line a metal sieve with a paper coffee filter. Set the sieve on top of a bowl that will hold about 1 cup of liquid. Place the contents of a pint of fat-free vanilla yogurt inside the paper-lined sieve and cover with plastic wrap or foil. Place the bowl in the refrigerator overnight. In the morning, liquid will have separated from the yogurt, reducing the volume to about half. This "cheese" is a fabulously healthy, protein-rich substitute for cream cheese and sour cream.
2. Cream the margarine and cream cheese with an electric mixer.
3. Add the sugar, salt, and almond extract; mix.
4. Add the egg whites, orange juice, orange zest, and flour; beat the mixture until smooth. Form the dough into a ball and chill it for 30 to 60 minutes.
5. After chilling the dough, preheat the oven to 350° Fahrenheit. Spray a 10" × 15" cookie sheet with olive-oil spray. Press the cookie dough evenly over the sheet.
6. Bake the crusts for 12 to 15 minutes, just until their edges are golden brown.
7. While the crusts are cooling, cream all the frosting ingredients together by hand or with a mixer.
8. Spread the crusts with the sauce/frosting mixture, then spread each type of fruit evenly over the sauce. Chill the tarts or serve them immediately. (Fruit is best at room temperature.)

Preparation time: 30 minutes (plus chilling time of 30 minutes)

Cooking time: 15 minutes

Nutrition Information per Serving:
277 calories, 4 g protein, 36 g carbohydrates, 1 g fiber,
13 g fat, 42% calories from fat, 0.08 mg vitamin B_6, 37 mcg folic acid,
48 mg calcium, 1 mg iron, 0 mg zinc

Strawberry Cheesecake

YIELD: 8 SERVINGS

Yes, you will see this on the menu for breakfast! It's so full of protein and cal-cium, and so low in fat, that it can be eaten any time of day. Don't tell any-one how healthy it is, and you can serve it for the fanciest dinner party. One more thing: Kris left off the crust because it just adds lots of fat and very few nutrients. You won't miss it!

8 ounces low-fat cream cheese, softened to room temperature
8 ounces fat-free cream cheese, softened to room temperature
32 ounces plain fat-free yogurt, made into yogurt cheese
    (See step 1 of the Orange Cream Fruit Tart recipe, page
    328, for how to make yogurt cheese. Just remember,
    you'll need to set the yogurt to drain overnight or 8 hours
    before making the recipe.)
4 egg whites
¾ cup plus 1 tablespoon sugar
1 tablespoon vanilla extract
3 tablespoons cornstarch
4 cups sliced strawberries

1. Preheat the oven to 350° Fahrenheit.
2. Combine all the ingredients, except strawberries, in a food proces-sor and blend them until smooth. Alternatively, combine all ingre-dients in a mixing bowl and use an electric mixer or mix by hand until smooth.
3. Spray a pie plate with the olive-oil spray. Pour the cheesecake mix-ture into the pie plate and bake it for 25 to 35 minutes, or until a knife inserted into its middle comes out clean.
4. Chill 2 hours or overnight.
5. Serve each slice of cheesecake with ½ cup of the strawberries.

Preparation time: 15 minutes, plus 2 hours chilling time

Cooking time: 25 to 35 minutes

Nutrition Information per Serving:
269 calories, 15 g protein, 42 g carbohydrates, 2 g fiber,
5 g fat, 17% calories from fat, 0.07 mg vitamin B_6, 20 mcg folic acid,
281 mg calcium, 1 mg iron, 1 mg zinc

Banana Smoothie

YIELD: 1 SERVING

Easy, delicious, and full of vitamin B$_6$!

> 1 banana
> ⅓ cup skim milk
> ¾ cup low-fat vanilla yogurt
> *Optional:* 1 cup ice cubes

1. Combine all ingredients in a food processor or blender; blend well.
2. You can add 1 cup of ice if you want a colder version; blend well.

Preparation time: 5 minutes

Cooking time: none

Nutrition Information per Serving:
294 calories, 13 g protein, 57 g carbohydrates, 3 g fiber,
3 g fat, 9% calories from fat, 0.80 mg vitamin B$_6$, 46 mcg folic acid,
422 mg calcium, 1 mg iron, 2 mg zinc

Chocolate Shake

YIELD: 1 SERVING

This shake is so thick and rich you'll think you're having something illegal!

    1 cup fat-free vanilla yogurt (not frozen yogurt)
    ½ cup chocolate sorbet

1. Place the ingredients in a blender.
2. Process them until smooth.

Preparation time: 5 minutes

Cooking time: none

Nutrition Information per Serving:
240 calories, 9 g protein, 52 g carbohydrates, 2 g fiber,
0 g fat, 0% calories from fat, 0 mg vitamin B_6, 0 mcg folic acid,
250 mg calcium, 0 mg iron, 0 mg zinc

Creamy Orange Shake

YIELD: 1 SERVING

This is one version of an orange shake that helps you meet folic acid requirements and tastes superb. Enjoy. If you're in a real hurry, just leave the vanilla out. Also, feel free to substitute fortified soy milk.

¼ cup orange juice concentrate, still frozen
1 cup skim milk
1 teaspoon vanilla extract

1. Combine all ingredients in a food processor or blender.
2. Process them until smooth.

Preparation time: 5 minutes

Cooking time: none

Nutrition Information per Serving:
205 calories, 9 g protein, 38 g carbohydrates, 1 g fiber,
1 g fat, 2% calories from fat, 0.20 mg vitamin B_6, 122 mcg folic acid,
302 mg calcium, 0.3 mg iron, 1 mg zinc

Double Raspberry Shake

YIELD: 1 SERVING

You'll be looking for this on the menu again and again!

½ cup raspberry sorbet
1 cup fresh or frozen raspberries
½ cup skim milk
3 tablespoons powdered skim milk

1. Combine all ingredients in a food processor or blender.
2. Process them until smooth.

Preparation time: 5 minutes

Cooking time: none

Nutrition Information per Serving:
258 calories, 10 g protein, 54 g carbohydrates, 8 g fiber,
1 g fat, 3% calories from fat, 0.16 mg vitamin B_6, 45 mcg folic acid,
335 mg calcium, 1 mg iron, 2 mg zinc

Frozen Chocolate Banana Shake

YIELD: 1 SERVING

Simply fabulous and so good for you and your baby! A delicious way to get vitamin B$_6$!

½ cup chocolate sorbet
¼ cup fat-free vanilla yogurt
1 banana

1. Combine all ingredients in a food processor or blender.
2. Process them until smooth.

Preparation time: 5 minutes

Cooking time: none

Nutrition Information per Serving:
272 calories, 5 g protein, 66 g carbohydrates, 5 g fiber,
0.6 g fat, 2% calories from fat, 0.68 mg vitamin B$_6$, 23 mcg folic acid,
90 mg calcium, 0.4 mg iron, 0.2 mg zinc

Frozen Lemonade

YIELD: 1 SERVING

A delicious and nutritious drink that is satisfying all year round.

8 ounces fat-free lemon yogurt (about 100 to 150 calories)
2 tablespoons powdered skim milk
3 tablespoons lemon juice
1 tablespoon honey
1 cup ice cubes

1. Combine all ingredients in a food processor or blender.
2. Process them until smooth.

Preparation time: 5 minutes

Cooking time: none

Nutrition Information per Serving:
236 calories, 11 g protein, 50 g carbohydrates, 0 g fiber,
0 g fat, 0% calories from fat, 0.06 mg vitamin B_6, 11 mcg folic acid,
359 mg calcium, 0.43 mg iron, 0.4 mg zinc

Karin's Banana Breakfast Frappé

YIELD: 1 SERVING

Another great way to get vitamin B$_6$ and calcium, and so easy.

> 1 cup skim milk
> 1 ripe banana
> 2 teaspoons honey
> *Optional*: 1 teaspoon vanilla extract

1. Combine all ingredients in food a processor or blender.
2. Process them until smooth.

Preparation time: 5 minutes

Cooking time: none

Nutrition Information per Serving:
249 calories, 10 g protein, 52 g carbohydrates, 3 g fiber,
1 g fat, 3% calories from fat, 0.78 mg vitamin B$_6$, 36 mcg folic acid,
310 mg calcium, 0.5 mg iron, 1 mg zinc

Peach Shake

YIELD: 1 SERVING

A delicious source of calcium and protein.

8 ounces fat-free peach yogurt
1 fresh peach, sliced (or ½ cup peaches canned in juice)
1 teaspoon honey
2 tablespoons powdered skim milk
1 cup ice cubes

1. Combine all ingredients in a blender or food processor.
2. Process them until smooth.

Preparation time: 5 minutes

Cooking time: none

Nutrition Information per Serving:
224 calories, 12 g protein, 45 g carbohydrates, 2 g fiber,
0 g fat, 1% calories from fat, 0.05 mg vitamin B_6, 8 mcg folic acid,
360 mg calcium, 0 mg iron, 1 mg zinc

Peanut Butter–Chocolate Shake

YIELD: 1 SERVING

This rich shake will satisfy your cravings for a peanut butter candy bar.

1 cup reduced-fat, vitamin enriched chocolate soymilk (or
    reduced-fat chocolate milk)
2 tablespoons smooth, natural peanut butter
3 ounces extra-firm light tofu (or ⅓ cup fat-free vanilla
    yogurt)

1. Place all ingredients in a blender or food processor.
2. Process them until smooth.

Preparation time: 5 minutes

Cooking time: none

Nutrition Information per Serving:

350 calories, 24 g protein, 21 g carbohydrates, 2 g fiber,
21 g fat, 51% calories from fat, 0.13 mg vitamin B_6, 86 mcg folic acid,
215 mg calcium, 1 mg iron, 1 mg zinc

Raspberry Banana Smoothie

YIELD: 1 SERVING

The raspberries and banana complement each other so well. We promise you that the tofu adds simply a creamy texture—no taste.

> 1 cup reduced-fat, vitamin-enriched soymilk (or skim milk)
> 1 banana
> 3 ounces extra-firm light tofu (or ⅓ cup fat-free vanilla
>   yogurt)
> ½ cup frozen raspberries
> 2 teaspoons honey

1. Place all ingredients in a blender.
2. Process them until smooth.

Preparation time: 5 minutes

Cooking time: none

Nutrition Information per Serving:

345 calories, 18 g protein, 60 g carbohydrates, 7 g fiber,

6 g fat, 14% calories from fat, 0.72 mg vitamin B_6, 78 mcg folic acid,

219 mg calcium, 1 mg iron, 1 mg zinc

Strawberry Milkshake

YIELD: 1 SERVING

When the urge for a milkshake strikes, you can satisfy it with this high-nutrition version. In fact, we recommend that you do.

> 1 cup skim milk
> 2 tablespoons powdered skim milk
> 2 teaspoons honey
> 2 cups frozen strawberries

1. Place all ingredients in a blender.
2. Process them until smooth.

Preparation time: 5 minutes

Cooking time: none

Nutrition Information per Serving:
258 calories, 13 g protein, 51 g carbohydrates, 8 g fiber,
2 g fat, 6% calories from fat, 0.33 mg vitamin B_6, 76 mcg folic acid,
453 mg calcium, 1.5 mg iron, 2 mg zinc

Vanilla Apricot Smoothie

YIELD: 1 SERVING

Kris's own personal favorite and a great way to get in those apricots that are so wonderfully nutritious.

3 apricots
½ cup fat-free vanilla yogurt
6 ounces light, firm tofu
¼ cup calcium fortified orange juice
Optional: 1 cup ice cubes

1. Combine all ingredients in a food processor or blender.
2. Process them until smooth.

Preparation time: 5 minutes

Cooking time: none

Nutrition Information per Serving:

188 calories, 16 g protein, 27 g carbohydrates, 2.5 g fiber,
1.8 g fat, 8% calories from fat, 0.09 mg vitamin B_6, 20 mcg folic acid,
275 mg calcium, 2 mg iron, 0.86 mg zinc

Hummus

Use this Middle Eastern dip in the Hummus Wrap (page 299) or for a delicious snack.

16 ounces garbanzo beans (drained)
3 tablespoons tahini (sesame butter; look for it in the
    ethnic foods section of your supermarket)
1 tablespoon lemon juice
½ teaspoon salt
1 clove garlic, chopped
¼ cup cold water
2 tablespoons olive oil
Optional: parsley and ground cayenne pepper for garnish

1. Place the garbanzo beans, tahini, lemon juice, salt, garlic, and water in a blender; purée the mixture until smooth.
2. Mix in the olive oil by hand; place the hummus in a serving dish or storage container. Garnish with snipped parsley and a pinch of ground cayenne pepper.

Preparation time: 10 minutes

Cooking time: none

Nutrition Information per Serving:
188 calories, 5 g protein, 15 g carbohydrates, 6 g fiber,
12 g fat, 56% calories from fat, 0.02 mg vitamin B_6, 9 mcg folic acid,
42 mg calcium, 2 mg iron, 1 mg zinc

Power Yogurt

YIELD: 1 SERVING

1 cup fat-free vanilla yogurt
3 tablespoons powdered skim milk
2 tablespoons dried cranberries (Craisins)
5 dates, chopped
2 tablespoons dried cherries
1 tablespoon almonds

1. Mix all ingredients into the yogurt.
2. Enjoy.

Preparation time: 5 minutes

Cooking time: none

Nutrition Information per Serving:
406 calories, 16 g protein, 77 g carbohydrates, 7 g fiber,
5 g fat, 11% calories from fat, 0.13 mg vitamin B_6, 17 mcg folic acid,
456 mg calcium, 1 mg iron, 1 mg zinc

A Note About Dried Fruit

You will see that dietitian Kristine Napier has used dried fruits in a number of recipes and meal plans, particularly in the third trimester. This is because when some of the water is taken out in the drying process, it makes the fruit a much more concentrated source of nutrients and calories. Although most people would be better off with fresh fruit, the third trimester fullness makes more nutrient- and calorie-dense foods like this very valuable. In other words, it is a lot easier to down four dried apricots than it is to fit in two fresh ones when you are already feeling full.

The problem with dried fruits is that many contain sulfur compounds as preservatives, and some contain sugar as an extra sweetener. Although tart dried cranberries would be inedible without the sugar, all other dried fruits are naturally sweet, so choose those that don't mention sugar in the ingredient list. The sulfur compounds used as preservatives provoke an allergic reaction in some people. If you are sensitive to these additives, choose dried fruits that don't contain them (check the label; you may need to go to a health-food store to find them) and keep the fruits in the refrigerator. Alternately, just substitute fresh fruits.

Trail Mix I

YIELD: 1 SERVING

2 tablespoons roasted soy nuts
2 tablespoons dried cranberries (Craisins)
2 tablespoons raisins
1 tablespoon semisweet chocolate chips

1. Combine all ingredients.
2. Enjoy.

Preparation time: 2 minutes

Cooking time: none

Nutrition Information per Serving:
209 calories, 5 g protein, 39 g carbohydrates, 3 g fiber,
6 g fat, 23% calories from fat, 0.09 mg vitamin B_6, 25 mcg folic acid,
28 mg calcium, 1 mg iron, 1 mg zinc

Trail Mixes . . . and More Trail Mixes

As you know by now, we want you to get more nuts and dried fruits into your diet for the minerals they supply. We've created three trail mix versions that are all about the same calorie level. Although we often specify one version or another because we are trying to fill out your nutrient intake on any given day, you can substitute one for another. Just make up a big batch of each to keep on hand.

Trail Mix II

YIELD: 1 SERVING

¼ cup Raisin Bran cereal
2 tablespoons almonds
3 tablespoons dried cherries

1. Combine all ingredients.
2. Enjoy.

Preparation time: 2 minutes

Cooking time: none

Nutrition Information per Serving:
207 calories, 5 g protein, 36 g carbohydrates, 6 g fiber,
9 g fat, 34% calories from fat, 0.26 mg vitamin B_6, 60 mcg folic acid,
55 mg calcium, 3 mg iron, 2 mg zinc

Trail Mix III

YIELD: 1 SERVING

¼ cup Fiber One cereal
3 tablespoons dried blueberries
2 tablespoons dried cranberries (Craisins)

1. Combine all ingredients.
2. Enjoy.

Preparation time: 2 minutes

Cooking time: none

Nutrition Information per Serving:
191 calories, 2 g protein, 48 g carbohydrates, 10 g fiber,
1 g fat, 6% calories from fat, 0.24 mg vitamin B_6, 11 mcg folic acid,
45 mg calcium, 4 mg iron, 1 mg zinc

Veggie Salsa Snack

YIELD: 1 SERVING

You can use any veggies you like; Kris chose this blend because they supply a great variety of nutrients.

Dip:
¼ cup fat-free sour cream
2 tablespoons favorite salsa

15 baby carrots
1 sweet bell pepper, sliced
3 stalks baby bok choy

1. Mix the sour cream and salsa.
2. Use it as dip for the veggies.

Preparation time: 5 minutes

Cooking time: none

Nutrition Information per Serving:
154 calories, 7 g protein, 31 g carbohydrates, 5 g fiber,
1 g fat, 6% calories from fat, 0.42 mg vitamin B_6, 99 mcg folic acid,
166 mg calcium, 2 mg iron, 0.5 mg zinc

CHAPTER ELEVEN

———————— 🍎 ————————

Remember, Life Outside the Womb Still Matters

You have embarked on one of the most precious jobs known to womankind: bringing a new life into the world. Indeed, it is an awesome responsibility. Although it has been clear for many years that during your pregnancy you act as the gatekeeper of your baby's good health, the new research on the early origins of chronic disease has revealed the startling information that a pregnant woman's diet and lifestyle may help to protect her child from illnesses that occur many decades after her birth. We all realize, however, that sometimes it is impossible to follow all nutrition guidelines to the letter, in spite of our best intentions. Certain medical conditions, such as an extreme form of morning sickness called hyperemesis gravidarum, can physically prevent our eating as well as we know we should during pregnancy. And even if you are physically perfect (if there is such a thing!), you may be aware of a genetic predisposition to certain health problems in your family.

As you'll recall, prenatal events may affect our children's risk of developing certain diseases, but those risks are definitely modified by how our children live their lives, including how they eat, how physically active they are, and whether they smoke. You can play an important role in explaining to your children early (and repeatedly) how important a healthy lifestyle and a healthy diet is, even in childhood and adolescence.

In this chapter, I would like to discuss briefly life outside the womb and how it impacts health, especially the conditions I discussed earlier in this book. The good news is it's never too late to change our diet, exercise, and other health habits to reduce our risks for disease. Fortunately, the advice for preventing most chronic diseases is very similar: When it comes to nutrition, exercise, and overall good health habits, the wellness program that reduces the risk of many types of cancer, for example, is much the same as the one that decreases our chances of developing heart disease, and as those that help to prevent high blood pressure, adult-onset diabetes, and obesity. We've put together the best advice from state-of-the-art research into one, easy-to-follow set of guidelines:

1. Maintain a healthfully lean body weight or drop excess pounds if you need to. To determine whether your weight is healthy, see pages 65 through 66. If you are concerned about your child's weight, speak with his or her pediatrician.

2. Cut back on your intake of high-fat foods, especially fried foods, fast foods, fatty meats, full-fat dairy foods, and fat-loaded bakery products and cookies—these foods are sources of saturated and *trans*-fats (see "About Fats," page 79, for more information on different types of fats). Similarly, avoid excessive sugars and refined carbohydrates, such as from soda, pastry or candy—these foods can add large amounts of calories without contributing nutrients to the diet and they can also hinder your metabolism.

3. Choose most of the foods you eat from plant sources, aiming to include each day:

   • At least nine servings (and preferably more) of fruits and vegetables (five servings for children) and five to seven servings of whole-grain foods (three to five for children)
   • At least one serving of legumes (dried beans, lentils, or peas) daily (a serving is ½ cup for adults, 2 tablespoons to ¼ cup for children)

4. Decrease total and low-density lipoprotein cholesterol (the bad cholesterol fraction) and increase high-density lipoprotein cholesterol (the good fraction). Do this by:

   • Decreasing your weight to an optimal scale reading
   • Replacing *trans*-fats and saturated fats with polyunsaturated and (preferably) monounsaturated fats, such as olive oil (refer to "About Fats" on page 79 for more information on different types of fat)

- Increasing your intake of fruits, vegetables, whole grains, and legumes
- Minimizing your dietary cholesterol intake
- Exercising regularly

5. If you eat meat, limit your intake of meat to 2 to 3 ounces twice per week, if possible. Instead, eat more fish and vegetable sources of protein, such as tofu and beans.

6. Increase your level of physical activity to at least 30 minutes per day on most (preferably all) days of the week.

7. Don't smoke. No matter what you tell your children about smoking, your actions speak louder than words. Set a good example by not smoking. Also, remember that secondhand smoke is extremely damaging to children's health.

8. Limit consumption of alcoholic beverages, if you drink at all.

LIFESTYLE ISSUES AND HEART DISEASE, HIGH BLOOD PRESSURE, CANCER, DIABETES, AND OBESITY

As we have learned, heart disease can result from being undernourished in the womb; we also know that atherosclerotic plaques—those fatty globs that clog arteries—can start forming as early as the preschool years. This is especially true when children eat a diet high in unhealthy fats, and even more so if they are too heavy. Although you can't change your age, your gender, or your genes, and although your disease risk may be affected by conditions in the womb, you can work on your modifiable risk factors from early childhood onward: being overweight, elevated cholesterol levels, high blood pressure, low physical activity, and smoking.

According to the National Heart, Lung, and Blood Institute, being overweight increases the chances of developing high blood pressure by two to six times. Similarly, people who are physically active have a lower risk of getting high blood pressure—a whopping 20% to 50% lower—than people who are not active. In addition to recommending managing these rather obvious factors, the National Heart, Lung, and Blood Institute also recommends reducing salt and sodium intake (the recommended maximum is about 2,400 milligrams sodium daily) and increasing your intake of foods rich in potassium, calcium, and magnesium, particularly fruits, vegetables, and whole-grain foods. Researchers suspect these minerals may be helpful in lowering blood pressure, based on recent results from the DASH Study (Dietary Approaches to Stop Hypertension).

What Is a Normal Blood Pressure?*

	Systolic (Upper) Reading (mm Hg)	Diastolic (Lower) Reading (mm Hg)
Normal	Less than 130	Less than 85
High normal	130–139	85–89
High blood pressure	Higher than 139	Higher than 89

Source: National Heart, Lung and Blood Institute, 2000.
*For adults over 18 years of age.

Adopting a healthy diet, exercise, and other healthy behaviors may also reduce your cancer risk by 30% to 40%, according to a report from the American Institute for Cancer Research and the World Cancer Research Fund. The American Cancer Society agrees: In May 2000, it announced the findings of a new research study indicating that women who ate the most foods recommended in current dietary guidelines were 30% less likely to die during the study follow-up period than study participants who consumed fewer of these "good foods." The American Cancer Society is especially concerned about the effects of lifestyle trends on the long-term health of children, who are establishing patterns of diet and exercise that may well last throughout their lifetimes. Undesirable trends include an increase in calories, a greater use of high-fat convenience foods, and a decline in physical activity. To combat these trends and reduce cancer risk, work toward adopting the dietary and lifestyle strategies recommended earlier.

The most important action we can take to reduce our risk for type 2 diabetes is to maintain a healthfully lean body weight, whether we're at increased risk because of a family history or certain fetal conditions. And in people who develop adult-onset diabetes, dropping excess weight can return blood sugars to normal.

Speaking of weight, the methods of avoiding gaining those extra pounds may seem so obvious that you wonder why we bothered to include them. On the other hand, if controlling excess weight were such a simple thing, we wouldn't find one third of the U.S. population battling obesity. As we discussed in Chapter Two, experts have several theories why certain conditions in the womb can increase the risk of obesity in later life. Avoiding these weight problems as an adult begins with establishing healthy eating patterns as a child. Here's what you can do to help your children:

- Foster a love for nature's bounty: Help your children learn to love vegetables by serving them at least twice a day. Serving vegetables as one of the main parts of the meal rather than as an afterthought is a great way to emphasize their importance. Mix up the colors, serving steamed, tender, brilliant-green broccoli with crisp, sweet carrot coins at lunch, for example. Your good example of enjoying these foods at lunch and dinner goes much further than you can imagine!

- Choose the best milk: Today, pediatricians are very clear about what kind of milk your children need. After the first year of life, young toddlers should have whole milk. Its protein–calorie–fat balance best meets the need of quickly growing children. After 2 years of age, your children should drink skim milk. Yes, even if your children seem to be thin or have trouble gaining weight, don't rely on the milkfat in whole milk. Instead, speak to their pediatrician about other foods to add to their diet. Just like learning to love vegetables later in life, it is very difficult for adolescents and adults to switch to skim milk when a love for 2% or whole milk is so well established.

- Mix up protein foods—and skimp on them. It is the American way to plan meals around protein food: mostly chicken, beef, and pork. It is also the American way to serve up oversize portions of these foods. Begin early to introduce your child to a wide variety of protein foods, as well as much smaller portions. To take the emphasis off meat, establish the habit of serving at least two vegetable sources of protein for dinner every week. Find recipes the whole family enjoys for black beans, tofu, split peas, and other beans and legumes. The advantage of vegetable sources of protein: You'll get the protein you're looking for in lots fewer calories and much less fat. As a bonus, many of these foods also provide extra fiber.

- Snack wisely. Exchange the cookie jar for a fruit bowl and a vegetable platter.

- Hold the liquid calories. Too many kids grow up quenching their thirst with soda and other sweet drinks, when a cool glass of water or skim milk (whole milk between ages 1 and 2 years) would do.

PARTING THOUGHTS

There are many factors that will influence your children's health through their adult life, some that you, as their mother, can influence, and some that you cannot. You cannot alter their genetic makeups, but you can prompt changes in their diets and exercise routines by explaining the reasons why, emphasizing the importance, and leading by good example. The one lifelong factor that you can influence right now, if you are already pregnant, or over the coming 9 months, if you are yet to conceive, is to provide your child with the best possible life in the womb. Simply by following an optimal diet (such as the Optimal Pregnancy Diet in this book) and adopting other healthy behaviors, you not only give your baby the best chance of being born healthy but also reduce his or her risk of diseases, ranging from certain types of cancer to diabetes to heart disease, many decades into the future.

Awareness of the importance of prenatal life places you, a mother-to-be of the early twenty-first century, at a new frontier in health care. This research, which is ongoing in many universities, hospitals, and research centers around the world, allows mothers to do more than ever before for their children. Imagine being able to influence your children's well-being for so long after they leave your womb. We never would have thought it possible just a few years ago.

I am so excited to be able to bring my and other scientists' results out of research institutions and to translate them into readable, usable information for women everywhere. Although I love the detective work my research entails, I recognize that the true victory is not in explaining the cause of a disease or other health problem but in using that information to help people to prevent the ailment. With *The Gift of Health,* I hope not only to help all mothers have as healthy babies as possible but also to improve the well-being of a whole generation of adults in four or five decades' time.

BIBLIOGRAPHY

BOOKS

Barker, D. J. P. *Fetal and Infant Origins of Adult Disease*. London: BMJ Publishing Group, 1992.

Barker, D. J. P. *Mothers, Babies, and Health in Later Life*. London: Churchill Livingstone, 1998.

Barker, D. J. P., ed. *Fetal Origins of Cardiovascular and Lung Disease*. New York: Marcel Dekker, 2000.

Kuh, D., Ben-Shlomo, Y., eds. *A Life Course Approach to Chronic Disease Epidemiology*. Oxford: Oxford Medical Publications, 1997.

Nathanielsz, P. W. *Life in the Womb: The Origin of Health and Disease*. Ithaca, NY: Promethean Press, 1999.

Susser, E. S., Gorman, J. M., Brown, A. S., eds. *Prenatal Exposures in Schizophrenia*. Washington, DC: American Psychiatric Press, 1999.

SCIENTIFIC PUBLICATIONS

Akre, O., Ekbom, A., Hsieh, C. C., et al. "Testicular nonseminoma and seminoma in relation to perinatal characteristics." *J Nat Cancer Inst* 1996; 88:883–9.

Barker, D. J. P., Winter, P. D., Osmond, C., et al. "Weight in infancy and death from ischaemic heart disease." *Lancet* 1989; ii:577–80.

Barker, D. J. "The fetal and infants origins of adult disease." *BMJ* 1990; 301:1111.

Barker, D. J. P., "Fetal origins of coronary heart disease." *BMJ* 1995; 311:171–4.

Barker, D. J. P., Gluckman, P. D., Godfrey, K. M., et al. "Fetal nutrition and cardiovascular disease in adult life." *Lancet* 1993; 341:938–41.

Barker, D. J. "In utero programming of cardiovascular disease." *Theriogenology* 2000; 53:555–74.

Barker, D. J., Shiell, A. W., Barker, M. E., et al. "Growth in utero and blood pressure levels in the next generation." *J Hypertens* 2000; 18:843–6.

Brown, A. S., Susser, E. S., Lin, S. P., et al. "Increased risk of affective disorders in males after second trimester prenatal exposure to the Dutch hunger winter of 1944–45." *Br J Psychiatry* 1995; 166:601–6.

Brown, A. S., Susser, E. S., Butler, P. D., et al. "Neurobiological plausibility of prenatal nutritional deprivation as a risk factor for schizophrenia." *J Nerv Ment Dis* 1996; 184:71–85.

Brown, L. M., Pottern, L. M., Hoover, R. N. "Prenatal and perinatal risk factors for testicular cancer." *Cancer Res* 1986; 46:4812–6.

Campbell, D. M., Hall, M. H., Barker, D. J., et al. "Diet in pregnancy and the offspring's blood pressure forty years later." *Br J Obstet Gynaecol* 1996; 103:273–80.

Clark, P. M., Atton, C., Law, C. M., et al. "Weight gain in pregnancy, triceps skinfold thickness, and blood pressure in offspring." *Obstet Gynecol.* 1998; 91:103–7.

Cnattingius, S., Zack, M. M., Ekbom, A., et al. "Prenatal and neonatal risk factors for childhood lymphatic leukemia." *J Nat Cancer Inst* 1995; 87:908–14.

Curhan, G. C., Chertow, G. M., Willett, W. C., et al. "Birth weight and adult hypertension and obesity in women." *Circulation* 1996; 94:1310–5.

Curhan, G. C, Willett, W. C, Rimm, E. B., et al. "Birth weight and adult hypertension, diabetes mellitus, and obesity in U.S. men." *Circulation* 1996; 94:3246–50.

Daling, J. R., Starzyk, P., Olshan, A., et al. "Birth weight and the incidence of childhood cancer." *J Natl Cancer Inst* 1984; 72:1039–41.

Ekbom, A., Trichopoulos, D., Adami, H. O., et al. "Evidence of prenatal influences on breast cancer risk." *Lancet* 1992; 340:1015–8.

Ekbom, A., Thurfjell, E., Hsieh, C. C., et al. "Perinatal characteristics and adult mammographic patterns." *Int J Cancer* 1995; 61:177–80.

Ekbom, A., Hsieh, C. C., Lipworth, L., et al. "Perinatal characteristics in relation to incidence of and mortality from prostate cancer." *BMJ* 1996; 313:337–41.

Ekbom, A., Hsieh, C. C., Lipworth, L., et al. "Intrauterine environment and breast cancer risk in women: a population-based study." *J Natl Cancer Inst* 1997; 88:71–6.

Ekbom, A. "Growing evidence that several human cancers may originate in utero." *Semin Cancer Biol* 1998; 8:237–44.

Fall, C. H. D., Osmond, C., Barker, D. J. P., et al. "Fetal and infant growth and cardiovascular risk factors in women." *BMJ* 1995; 310:428–32.

Forsén, T. J., Eriksson, J. G., Tuomilehto, J., et al. "Mother's weight in pregnancy and coronary heart disease in a cohort of Finnish men: follow up study." *BMJ* 1997; 315:837–40.

Forsén, T., Eriksson, J. G., Tuomilehto, J., et al. "Growth in utero and during childhood among women who develop coronary heart disease: longitudinal study." *BMJ* 1999; 319:1403–7.

Forsén, T., Eriksson, J., Tuomilehto, J., et al. "The fetal and childhood growth of persons who develop type 2 diabetes." *Ann Intern Med* 2000; 133:176–82.

Frischer, T., Kuehr, J., Meinert, R., et al. "Relationship between low birth weight and respiratory symptoms in a cohort of primary school children." *Acta Paediatr* 1992; 81:1040–1.

Godfrey, K. M., Forrester, T., Barker, D. J. P., et al. "Maternal nutritional status in pregnancy and blood pressure in childhood." *Br J Obstet Gynaecol* 1994; 101:398–403.

Godfrey, K. M., Barker, D. J. "Fetal nutrition and adult disease." *Am J Clin Nutr* 2000; 71(5 Suppl):1344S–52S.

Godfrey, K. M., Robinson, S., Baker, D. J. P., et al. "Maternal nutrition in early and late pregnancy in relation to placental and fetal growth." *Br Med J* 1996; 312:410–4.

Gold, E., Gordis, L., Tonascia, J., et al. "Risk Factors for Brain Tumors in Children." *Am J Epidemiol* 1979; 109:309–19.

Hagstrom, B., Nyberg, P., Nilsoon, P. M. "Asthma in adult life—is there an association with birth weight?" *Scand J Prim Health Care* 1998; 16:117–20.

Harding, J. E. "The nutritional basis of the fetal origins of adult disease." *Int J Epidemiol* 2001 (in press).

Hilakivi-Clarke, L., Onojafe, I., Raygada, M., et al. "Breast cancer risk in rats fed a diet high in n-6 polyunsaturated fatty acids during pregnancy." *J Natl Cancer Inst* 1996; 88:1821–7.

Hilakivi-Clarke, L., Clarke, R., Onojafe, I., et al. "A maternal diet high in n-6 polyunsaturated fats alters mammary gland development, puberty onset, and breast cancer risk among female rat offspring." *Proc Natl Acad Sci USA* 1997; 94:9372–7.

Hilakivi-Clarke, L., Stoica, A., Raygada, M., et al. "Consumption of a high-fat diet alters estrogen receptor content, protein kinase C activity, and mammary gland morphology in virgin and pregnant mice and female offspring." *Cancer Res* 1998; 58:654–60.

Hilakivi-Clarke, L., Clarke, R., Lippman, M. "The influence of maternal diet on breast risk among female offspring." *Nutrition* 1999; 15:392–401.

Hoek, H. W., Susser, E., Buck, K. A., et al. "Schizoid personality disorder after prenatal exposure to famine." *Am J Psychiatry* 1996; 153:1637–9.

Kitchen, W. H., Olinsky, A., Doyle, L. W., et al. "Respiratory Health and Lung Function in Eight-Year-Old Children of Very Low Birth Weight: A Cohort Study." *Pediatrics* 1992; 89:1151–8.

Law, C. M., de Swiet, M., Osmond, C., et al. "Initiation of hypertension in utero and its amplification throughout life." *BMJ* 1993; 306:24–7.

Law, C. M., Gordon, G. S., Shiell, A. W. "Thinness at birth and glucose tolerance in seven-year-old children." *Diabet Med* 1995; 12:24–9.

Leadbitter, P., Pearce, N., Cheng, S., et al. "Relationship between fetal growth and the development of asthma and atopy in childhood." *Thorax* 1999; 54:905–10.

Leon, D. A., Koupilova, I., Lithell, H. O., et al. "Failure to realise growth potential in utero and adult obesity in relation to blood pressure in fifty-year-old Swedish men." *BMJ* 1996; 312:401–6.

Leon, D. A., Lithell, H. O., Vågerö, D., et al. "Reduced fetal growth rate and increased risk of death from ischaemic heart disease: cohort study of 15,000 Swedish men and women born 1915–29." *BMJ* 1998; 317:241–5.

Lewis, S., Richards, D., Bynner, J., et al. "Prospective study of risk factors for early and persistent wheezing in childhood." *Eur Respir J* 1995; 8:349–56.

Lithell, H. O., McKeigue, P. M., Berglund, L., et al. "Relation of size at birth to non-insulin dependent diabetes and insulin concentrations in men aged fifty to sixty years." *BMJ* 1996; 312:406–10.

Lopuhaä, C. E., Roseboom, T. J., Osmond, C., et al. "Atopy, lung function and obstructive airways disease in adults after prenatal exposure to famine." *Thorax* 2000; 55:555–61.

Lumey, L. H., Ravelli, A. C. J., Wiessing, L. G., et al. "The Dutch famine birth cohort study: design, validation of exposure, and selected characteristics of subjects after forty-three years follow-up." *Paediatr Perinat Epidemiol* 1993; 7:354–67.

MacMahon, B., Newill, V. A. "Birth characteristics of children dying of malignant neoplasms." *J Nat Cancer Inst* 1962; 28:231–44.

Martyn, C. N., Barker, D. J. P., Jespersen, S., et al. "Growth in utero, adult blood pressure, and arterial compliance." *Br Heart J* 1995; 73:116–21.

Martyn, C. N., Hales, C. N., Barker, D. J., et al. "Fetal growth and hyperinsulinaemia in adult life." *Diabet Med* 1998; 15:688–94.

McCredite, M., Maisonneuve, P., Boyle, P. "Antenatal risk factors for malignant brain tumours in New South Wales children." *Int J Cancer* 1994; 56:6–10.

Michels, K. B., Trichopoulos, D., Robins, J. M., et al. "Birthweight as a risk factor for breast cancer." *Lancet* 1996; 348:1542–6.

Michels, K. B., Trichopoulos, D., Rosner, B. A., et al. "Being breastfed in infancy and breast cancer incidence in adult life: results from the two Nurses' Health Studies." *Am J Epidemiol* 2001; 153:275–83.

Mi, J., Law, C., Zhang, K. L., et al. "Effects of infant birthweight and maternal body mass index in pregnancy on components of insulin resistance syndrome in China." *Ann Intern Med* 2000; 132:253–60.

Neugebauer, R., Hoek, H. W., Susser, E. "Prenatal exposure to wartime famine and development of antisocial personality disorder in early adulthood." *JAMA* 1999; 282:455–62.

Osmond, C., Barker, D. J. "Fetal, infant, and childhood growth are predictors of coronary heart disease, diabetes, and hypertension in adult men and women." *Environ Health Perspect* 2000; 108 Suppl 3:545–53.

Petridou, E., Koussouri, M., Toupadaki, N., et al. "Diet during pregnancy and risk of cerebral palsy." *Br J Nutr* 1998; 79:407–12.

Preston-Martin, S., Pogoda, J. M., Mueller, B. A., et al. "Maternal consumption of cured meats and vitamins in relation to pediatric brain tumors." *Cancer Epidemiol Biomarkers Prev* 1996; 5:599–605.

Ravelli, G. P., Stein, Z. A., Susser, M. W. "Obesity in young men after famine exposure *in utero* and early infancy." *N Engl J Med* 1976; 295:349–53.

Ravelli, A. C. J., van der Meulen, J. H. P., Michels, R. P. J., et al. "Glucose tolerance in adults after prenatal exposure to famine." *Lancet* 1998; 351:173–77.

Ravelli, A. C., van Der Meulen, J. H., Osmond, C., et al. "Obesity at the age of fifty in men and women exposed to famine prenatally." *Am J Clin Nutr* 1999; 70:811–6.

Rich-Edwards, J. W., Stampfer, M. J., Manson, J. E., et al. "Birth weight and risk of cardiovascular disease in a cohort of women followed up since 1976." *BMJ* 1997; 315:396–400.

Rich-Edwards, J. W., Colditz, G. A., Stampfer, M. J., et al. "Birthweight and the risk for type 2 diabetes mellitus in adult women." *Ann Intern Med* 1999; 130:278–84.

Roseboom, T. J., van Der Meulen, J. H., Osmond, C., et al. "Coronary heart disease after prenatal exposure to the Dutch famine, 1944–45." *Heart* 2000; 84:595–8.

Roseboom, T. J., van Der Meulen, J. H., Osmond, C., et al. "Plasma lipid profiles in adults after prenatal exposures to the Dutch famine." *Am J Clin Nutr* 2000; 72:1101–6.

Ross, J. A., Potter, J. D., Shu, X. O., et al. "Evaluating the relationships among maternal reproductive history, birth characteristics, and infant leukemia: a report from the Children's Cancer Group." *Ann Epidemiol* 1997; 7:172–9.

Sabroe, S., Olsen, J. "Perinatal correlates of specific histological types of testicular cancer in patients below thirty-five years of age: a case-cohort study based on midwives' records in Denmark." *Int J Cancer* 1998; 78:140–3.

Sanderson, M., Williams, M. A., Malone, K. E., et al. "Perinatal factors and risk of breast cancer." *Epidemiology* 1996; 7:34–7.

Schaefer, C. A., Brown, A. S., Wyatt, R. J., et al. "Maternal prepregnant body mass and risk of schizophrenia in adult offspring." *Schizophr Bull* 2000; 26:275–86.

Schwartz, J., Gold, D., Dockery, D. W., et al. "Predictors of asthma and persistent wheeze in a national sample of children in the United States." *Am Rev Respir Dis* 1990; 142:555–62.

Schymura, M. J., Zheng, D., Baptiste, M. S., et al. "A case-control study of childhood brain tumors and maternal lifestyle." *Am J Epidemiol* 1996; 143:S8.

Shaheen, S. O., Sterne, J. A., Montgomery, S. M., et al. "Birth weight, body mass index and asthma in young adults." *Thorax* 1999; 54:396–402.

Shiell, A. W., Campbell, D. M., Hall, M. H., et al. "Diet in late pregnancy and glucose-insulin metabolism of the offspring forty years later." *Br J Obstet Gynaecol* 2000; 107:890–5.

Sørensen, H. T., Sabroe, S., Olsen, J., et al. "Birth weight and cognitive function in young adult life: historical cohort study." *BMJ* 1997; 315:401–3.

Stein, C. E., Fall, C. H. D., Kumaran, K., et al. "Fetal growth and coronary heart disease in South India." *Lancet* 1996; 348:1269–73.

Susser, E. S., Lin, S. P. "Schizophrenia after prenatal exposure to the Dutch Hunger Winter of 1944–1945." *Arch Gen Psychiatry* 1992; 49:983–8.

Susser, E. B., Brown, A., Matte, T. D. "Prenatal factors and adult mental and physical health." *Can J Psychiatry* 1999; 44:326–34.

Tibblin, G., Eriksson, M., Cnattingius, S., et al. "High birthweight as a predictor of prostate cancer risk." *Epidemiology* 1995; 6:423–4.

Trichopoulos, D. "Hypothesis: does breast cancer originate in utero?" *Lancet* 1990; 335:939–40.

Westergaard, T., Andersen, P. K., Pedersen, J. B., et al. "Birth characteristics, sibling patterns, and acute leukemia risk in childhood: a population-based cohort study." *J Nat Cancer Inst* 1997; 89:939–47.

Index